The Impact of Malaria on the Social-Economic Development of West Africa

Mogana S. Flomo, Jr.

Published by MGI Inc., 2023.

THE IMPACT OF MALARIA ON THE SOCIAL-ECONOMIC DEVELOPMENT OF WEST AFRICA

First edition. July 19, 2023.

Copyright © 2023 Mogana S. Flomo, Jr..

ISBN: 979-8223380160

Written by Mogana S. Flomo, Jr..

Table of Contents

Dedication

Malaria remains a formidable global health challenge, particularly in West Africa, where it continues to impede socio-economic development. This book examines the impact of malaria on the region, focusing on prevalence, health consequences, productivity losses, and social implications. It identifies the most affected countries and regions, emphasizing the factors that contribute to high transmission rates. The book investigates the health consequences of malaria, specifically its effect on mortality rates among children and pregnant women, as well as the long-term implications of recurring infections on individual health and well-being. Furthermore, it explores the economic ramifications, including productivity losses, agricultural and food security concerns, healthcare costs, and indirect expenses related to education and tourism. The social consequences of malaria, such as stigma and discrimination, are discussed, along with an examination of the disease's gender dimensions. The book provides an overview of existing malaria control interventions, analyzes their challenges and limitations, and investigates innovative strategies and technologies for malaria control in the region. Additionally, it explores international efforts, highlighting key initiatives such as the Roll Back Malaria Partnership and the Global Fund to Fight AIDS, Tuberculosis, and Malaria. The importance of collaboration between governments, NGOs, and the private sector is underscored. The book identifies countries or regions that have made significant progress in malaria control and investigates the factors contributing to their success. Finally, it draws lessons learned and presents policy recommendations for improving malaria control strategies. The book advocates for increased investment in research, healthcare infrastructure, and capacity building to combat malaria effectively and promote sustainable socio-economic development in West Africa.

Description

Malaria remains a formidable global health challenge, particularly in West Africa, where it continues to impede socio-economic development. This book examines the impact of malaria on the region, focusing on prevalence, health consequences, productivity losses, and social implications. It identifies the most affected countries and regions, emphasizing the factors that contribute to high transmission rates. The book investigates the health consequences of malaria, specifically its effect on mortality rates among children and pregnant women, as well as the long-term implications of recurring infections on individual health and well-being. Furthermore, it explores the economic ramifications, including productivity losses, agricultural and food security concerns, healthcare costs, and indirect expenses related to education and tourism. The social consequences of malaria, such as stigma and discrimination, are discussed, along with an examination of the disease's gender dimensions. The book provides an overview of existing malaria control interventions, analyzes their challenges and limitations, and investigates innovative strategies and technologies for malaria control in the region. Additionally, it explores international efforts, highlighting key initiatives such as the Roll Back Malaria Partnership and the Global Fund to Fight AIDS, Tuberculosis, and Malaria. The importance of collaboration between governments, NGOs, and the private sector is underscored. The book identifies countries or regions that have made significant progress in malaria control and investigates the factors contributing to their success. Finally, it draws lessons learned and presents policy recommendations for improving malaria control strategies. The book advocates for increased investment in research, healthcare infrastructure, and capacity building to combat malaria effectively and promote sustainable socio-economic development in West Africa.

Acronyms

ACT - Artemisinin-Based Combination Therapy
ANC - Antenatal Care
ARDS - Acute Respiratory Distress Syndrome
EIR - Entomological Inoculation Rate
G6PD - Glucose-6-Phosphate Dehydrogenase
HRP2 - Histidine-Rich Protein 2
IPT - Intermittent Preventive Treatment
IPTi - Intermittent Preventive Treatment in Infants
IPTp - Intermittent Preventive Treatment during Pregnancy
IRS - Indoor Residual Spraying
ITN - Insecticide-Treated Net
ITNs - Insecticide-Treated Nets
LLINs - Long-lasting Insecticidal Nets
NGO - Non-Governmental Organization
PCR - Polymerase Chain Reaction
RDT - Rapid Diagnostic Test
RDTs - Rapid Diagnostic Tests
SP - Sulfadoxine-Pyrimethamine
USD - United States Dollar
WHO - World Health Organization

Chapter 1. Introduction

1.1 Brief overview of malaria as a global health issue

Malaria is a life-threatening disease caused by the Plasmodium parasite and transmitted through the bites of infected female Anopheles mosquitoes. It poses a significant global health burden, particularly in tropical and subtropical regions. According to the World Health Organization (WHO), an estimated 229 million cases of malaria occurred worldwide in 2019, leading to approximately 409,000 deaths, mostly among children under the age of five.

Malaria is prevalent in many parts of the world, with sub-Saharan Africa bearing the highest burden. In this region, over 90% of malaria cases and deaths occur, affecting primarily young children and pregnant women. The disease has a profound impact on socio-economic development, exacerbating poverty and hindering progress in affected countries.

Efforts to combat malaria have been ongoing for decades, focusing on various strategies such as vector control, access to early diagnosis and treatment, and research for new tools and interventions. International partnerships and organizations, including the WHO, have played a crucial role in coordinating and supporting global malaria control initiatives.

Despite progress in recent years, malaria remains a significant public health challenge, particularly in regions like West Africa. Understanding the impact of malaria on the socio-economic development of this specific region is essential for formulating effective interventions and policies to mitigate its effects.

1.2 Focus on the prevalence and impact of malaria in West Africa

West Africa is one of the most malaria-endemic regions in the world, experiencing a high burden of the disease. Malaria transmission in this region is primarily caused by Plasmodium falciparum, the most severe and deadly species of the parasite. The prevalence and impact of malaria in West Africa have far-reaching consequences on the health and socio-economic development of the affected countries.

1.2.1 Prevalence of Malaria:

1. ***High transmission*** rates: West Africa experiences intense and perennial malaria transmission, with transmission occurring throughout the year in many areas.
2. ***Substantial malaria burden***: The region accounts for a significant proportion of global malaria cases and deaths. It is estimated that West Africa contributes to over 70% of malaria cases and deaths in Africa.

1.2.2 Health Impact of Malaria:

1. **High mortality rates:** Malaria-related deaths are most prevalent among children under five years of age. West Africa has witnessed a considerable number of malaria-related deaths, leading to increased child mortality rates.

2. *Morbidity and illness:* Malaria causes frequent episodes of fever, fatigue, and other debilitating symptoms, leading to reduced productivity and economic losses. c. Vulnerability of pregnant women: Malaria infection during pregnancy poses significant risks to both the mother and the unborn child, increasing the likelihood of maternal anemia, low birth weight, and infant mortality.

1.2.3 Economic Impact of Malaria:

1. ***Productivity losses***: Malaria-related illnesses and deaths result in significant productivity losses due to missed workdays, reduced agricultural output, and decreased economic activities.
2. ***Healthcare costs***: The economic burden of malaria includes direct healthcare expenditures for diagnosis, treatment, and prevention, placing a strain on already limited healthcare budgets.
3. ***Educational impact***: Malaria affects school attendance and performance, leading to reduced educational attainment and hindering human capital development.
4. ***Impaired tourism and investment***: Malaria prevalence in West Africa discourages tourism and foreign investments, affecting economic growth and development.

1.2.4 Social Impact of Malaria:

1. ***Stigma and discrimination***: Malaria is often associated with poverty and lack of proper healthcare, leading to stigmatization of affected individuals and communities.
2. ***Gender disparities***: Malaria disproportionately affects women and girls, influencing their access to education, employment opportunities, and overall social well-being.
3. ***Disruption of social structures***: Malaria can disrupt social cohesion, community development, and resilience, as affected individuals and communities face repeated health and economic challenges.

Understanding the prevalence and impact of malaria in West Africa is crucial for policymakers, healthcare providers, and researchers to develop targeted interventions and allocate resources effectively. By addressing the specific challenges posed by malaria in this region, efforts can be focused on improving health outcomes and promoting sustainable socio-economic development.

1.3 Objectives of this book:

This book aims to explore the impact of malaria on the socio-economic development of West African countries.

In this book, we will comprehensively examine the multifaceted impact of malaria on the socio-economic development of West African countries. By analyzing the prevalence of malaria, its health consequences, and the resulting economic and social implications, we aim to shed light on the challenges faced by these nations in achieving sustainable development. Through a thorough evaluation of existing control and prevention strategies, international partnerships, and successful case studies, we will provide insights and recommendations for mitigating the detrimental effects of malaria and promoting socio-economic progress in West Africa.

Chapter 2. Epidemiology of Malaria in West Africa

2.1 Statistics on the prevalence and burden of malaria in West Africa

Malaria continues to be a significant public health concern in West Africa, with the region bearing a substantial burden of the disease. The following statistics highlight the prevalence and impact of malaria in West African countries:

2.1.1 High malaria burden:

The high malaria burden in West Africa is a significant public health challenge with profound implications for the region. The statistics provided by the World Health Organization (WHO) emphasize the extent of this burden:

According to the WHO (2020), West Africa contributes to over 70% of malaria cases and deaths in Africa. This statistic highlights the disproportionate burden of malaria in the region compared to other parts of the continent. With West Africa accounting for more than two-thirds of malaria cases and deaths in Africa, it underscores the urgency and critical need for effective malaria control measures in this area.

Furthermore, the WHO (2020) estimates that over 90% of the West African population lives in areas at risk of malaria transmission. This estimate emphasizes the widespread vulnerability of the population in West Africa to malaria. It indicates that the majority of people in the region reside in areas where the risk of malaria transmission is significant.

These statistics serve as a call to action, highlighting the urgent need for comprehensive and sustained efforts to combat malaria in West Africa. Effective interventions, such as the distribution of insecticide-treated bed nets, indoor residual spraying, access to accurate diagnosis and effective treatment, as well as community education and engagement, are crucial in reducing the malaria burden (WHO, 2020).

Addressing the high malaria burden in West Africa through targeted interventions and comprehensive strategies will not only improve the health and well-being of the population but also contribute to broader socio-economic development in the region. By prioritizing malaria control and prevention, West African countries can make significant strides in reducing the impact of malaria and improving the lives of their populations (WHO, 2020).

2.1.2 Malaria cases and deaths:

The high malaria burden in West Africa is a significant public health challenge with profound implications for the region. The statistics provided by the World Health Organization (WHO) emphasize the extent of this burden:

In 2019, an estimated 210 million malaria cases occurred in the African region, with a large proportion concentrated in West Africa (WHO, 2020) [1]. This staggering number highlights the significant burden of malaria in the region. West Africa, with its high prevalence of malaria cases, plays a major role in contributing to the overall malaria burden on the continent.

Furthermore, the number of malaria-related deaths in West Africa is significant, with the region accounting for a substantial proportion of malaria deaths globally (WHO, 2020). The exact figures may vary from year to year, but the impact of malaria-related deaths in West Africa remains a critical concern.

These statistics serve as a stark reminder of the urgent need for effective malaria control measures in West Africa. The burden of malaria on the region's health systems, economies, and communities is substantial. It is imperative to implement comprehensive and sustained efforts to combat malaria and reduce its impact on the population.

Addressing the high malaria burden in West Africa through targeted interventions and comprehensive strategies is crucial. By prioritizing malaria control and prevention, West African countries can make significant strides in reducing the number of malaria cases and deaths. Implementation of strategies such as widespread distribution of insecticide-treated bed nets, indoor residual spraying, access to accurate diagnosis, and effective treatment are key components of malaria control programs in the region.

In conclusion, the high malaria burden in West Africa, characterized by a large number of malaria cases and significant malaria-related deaths, underscores the urgent need for intensified efforts in malaria control. Effective interventions and strategies, guided by evidence-based practices, can contribute to reducing the burden of malaria and improving the health and well-being of the population in West Africa.

2.1.3 Malaria prevalence:

The prevalence of malaria in West Africa is a significant concern, with variations observed across countries and regions within the region. The World Health Organization (WHO) provides key insights into malaria prevalence in West Africa:

Malaria transmission in West Africa is primarily caused by the Plasmodium falciparum parasite, which is responsible for the most severe form of the disease (WHO, 2020). Plasmodium falciparum is known for its high morbidity and mortality rates, particularly among vulnerable populations such as children and pregnant women.

The prevalence of malaria varies across countries and regions within West Africa, with some areas experiencing high and perennial transmission (WHO, 2020). Factors such as climate, ecological conditions, and the presence of suitable mosquito vectors contribute to the varying levels of malaria transmission. Some regions may have consistent and intense transmission throughout the year, while others may experience seasonal fluctuations in malaria prevalence.

These findings highlight the complex nature of malaria transmission in West Africa. The predominance of Plasmodium falciparum and the varying levels of malaria prevalence underscore the need for tailored and context-specific malaria control strategies.

Addressing malaria prevalence in West Africa requires a multi-faceted approach. It includes interventions such as the distribution of insecticide-treated bed nets, indoor residual spraying, access to prompt and accurate diagnosis, and effective treatment. Additionally, targeted efforts should focus on high transmission areas and vulnerable populations to achieve maximum impact in reducing malaria prevalence.

2.1.4 Impact on vulnerable populations:

Malaria has a disproportionate impact on vulnerable populations in West Africa, especially children under the age of five and pregnant women. The World Health Organization (WHO) provides insights into the vulnerability of these groups:

Children under the age of five are particularly vulnerable to malaria in West Africa (WHO, 2020). Their immature immune systems make them more susceptible to infection and severe complications. Malaria poses a significant threat to this age group, leading to increased morbidity and mortality rates.

Malaria is a leading cause of death among children under five in the region, contributing to high child mortality rates (WHO, 2020). The disease can rapidly progress in young children, leading to severe complications such as severe anemia, respiratory distress, and cerebral malaria. These complications, if left untreated, can result in death.

Pregnant women also face heightened vulnerability to malaria in West Africa (WHO, 2020). Pregnancy alters the immune response, making women more susceptible to infection and increasing the risk of adverse outcomes. Malaria in pregnancy can lead to maternal anemia, low birth weight, preterm birth, and neonatal mortality.

These findings highlight the critical need to prioritize malaria prevention and control strategies specifically targeted at protecting children under five and pregnant women in West Africa.

To address the impact on vulnerable populations, interventions such as the distribution of insecticide-treated bed nets and intermittent preventive treatment in pregnancy (IPTp) should be implemented. Insecticide-treated bed nets provide physical protection from mosquito bites, reducing the risk of infection for both children and pregnant women. IPTp involves the administration of antimalarial medication to pregnant women during routine antenatal care visits, offering protection against malaria during pregnancy.

Ensuring access to prompt and accurate diagnosis and effective treatment for children and pregnant women is essential. Early detection and treatment of malaria in these vulnerable groups can significantly reduce morbidity and mortality rates.

2.1.5 Economic burden:

Malaria imposes a substantial economic burden on West African countries, manifesting in productivity losses and increased healthcare expenditures. The World Health Organization (WHO) provides evidence of the economic impact of malaria:

Malaria's economic burden stems from various factors, including treatment costs, prevention measures, and loss of workdays (WHO, 2020). The expenses associated with malaria treatment, such as diagnostic tests, antimalarial drugs, and hospitalization, contribute to the rising healthcare expenditures in affected countries. These costs place a strain on healthcare systems and can lead to financial hardships for individuals and families.

Productivity losses are a significant component of the economic burden of malaria. The disease causes individuals to miss workdays due to illness, leading to reduced productivity in various sectors (WHO, 2020). The impact is particularly felt in industries such as agriculture, where a large portion of the workforce is engaged. Absenteeism and reduced work capacity due to malaria directly affect productivity levels and hinder economic growth.

The cumulative economic burden of malaria has adverse effects on the overall economies of affected countries. The costs associated with treatment, prevention, and productivity losses contribute to a decrease in national income and hinder socio-economic development. The diversion of resources to address malaria-related expenses also limits investments in other vital sectors.

Addressing the economic burden of malaria requires comprehensive strategies that focus on both prevention and treatment. Investing in cost-effective interventions, such as the distribution of insecticide-treated bed nets and the use of effective antimalarial drugs, can help reduce the incidence of malaria and subsequent economic costs.

Furthermore, improving access to healthcare services and ensuring prompt and accurate diagnosis and treatment contribute to reducing the economic burden. By addressing the underlying factors that hinder productivity, such as providing access to quality healthcare and implementing workplace malaria prevention measures, countries can mitigate the economic impact of malaria.

2.1.6 Regional variations:

Regional variations in malaria prevalence and burden exist within West Africa, with some countries experiencing higher transmission rates and greater health and economic impact compared to others. The World Health Organization (WHO) provides insights into these regional variations:

Countries such as Nigeria, Ghana, Burkina Faso, and Mali have been identified as high-burden countries with significant malaria-related challenges (WHO, 2020). These countries bear a substantial malaria burden, characterized by high prevalence rates, increased morbidity and mortality, and significant socio-economic consequences. Factors such as climate, geographical location, population density, and access to healthcare services contribute to the varying levels of malaria burden within these countries.

For example, Nigeria has one of the highest malaria burdens globally, with a high number of cases and deaths reported each year. The country faces challenges related to inadequate access to healthcare services, limited availability of diagnostic tools and effective treatment, and suboptimal use of preventive measures. Ghana, Burkina Faso, and Mali also grapple with significant malaria burdens, highlighting the need for targeted interventions and resource allocation in these areas.

Understanding the regional variations in malaria prevalence and burden is crucial for designing effective control and prevention strategies. Tailoring interventions to specific contexts and challenges allows for targeted allocation of resources and implementation of measures that address the unique needs of each country within West Africa.

By identifying high-burden countries and understanding the specific challenges they face, policymakers and public health authorities can prioritize resources and interventions in areas where the malaria burden is most significant. This targeted approach can lead to improved access to preventive measures, accurate diagnosis, effective treatment, and implementation of vector control strategies.

In conclusion, regional variations in malaria prevalence and burden exist within West Africa. High-burden countries such as Nigeria, Ghana, Burkina Faso, and Mali face significant challenges related to malaria control and prevention. By recognizing these variations and tailoring interventions to specific regional contexts, policymakers can allocate resources effectively and implement targeted strategies to reduce the socio-economic impact of malaria in West Africa.

. . . .

TABLE 1: SUMMARY INFORMATION on the prevalence and burden of malaria in West Africa

Statistics	Summary
High malaria burden	West Africa accounts for over 70% of malaria cases and deaths in Africa.
Malaria cases and deaths	West Africa contributes significantly to the estimated 210 million malaria cases in Africa.
Malaria prevalence	Malaria transmission is primarily caused by the Plasmodium falciparum parasite.
Impact on vulnerable populations	Children under five and pregnant women are particularly vulnerable to malaria in West Africa.
Economic burden	Malaria imposes a substantial economic burden through healthcare expenditures and productivity losses.
Regional variations	Countries such as Nigeria, Ghana, Burkina Faso, and Mali have higher malaria burdens.

The table provides a summary of key statistics on the prevalence and burden of malaria in West Africa, including the high malaria burden in the region, the number of malaria cases and deaths, variations in malaria prevalence, the impact on vulnerable populations, and the economic burden associated with the disease. It highlights the urgent need for effective interventions and targeted strategies to combat malaria and reduce its impact on the population and economies of West African countries.

23

2.2 The most affected countries and regions

Malaria is a major health concern in several countries and regions within West Africa. The following discussion highlights some of the most affected areas, supported by relevant in-text citations:

2.2.1 Nigeria:

Nigeria bears the highest malaria burden in West Africa, accounting for approximately 25% of global malaria cases (WHO, 2020). This statistic underscores the significant impact of malaria in the country and highlights the urgent need for effective control measures. The prevalence of malaria transmission is widespread throughout Nigeria, with all states considered at risk (WHO, 2020). This implies that the entire population is potentially exposed to malaria infection, emphasizing the need for comprehensive prevention and control strategies.

Regional variations within Nigeria contribute to differing malaria prevalence and burden. The northern regions of Nigeria, in particular, experience higher malaria prevalence and burden compared to the southern regions (Noland et al., 2020). Factors such as climate, ecological conditions, and socioeconomic factors contribute to these regional disparities. The northern regions, characterized by higher temperatures and more favorable breeding conditions for mosquitoes, face greater challenges in controlling malaria transmission.

Understanding these regional variations is crucial for implementing targeted interventions and allocating resources effectively. In the case of Nigeria, efforts should focus on the northern regions where malaria burden is highest. These interventions may include the distribution of insecticide-treated bed nets, access to prompt and accurate diagnosis and treatment, and implementation of vector control strategies.

To address the malaria burden in Nigeria, comprehensive approaches should consider the unique challenges and characteristics of each region. Collaborative efforts between the government, public health agencies, non-governmental organizations, and local communities are vital in implementing and sustaining effective malaria control programs.

In conclusion, Nigeria bears the highest malaria burden in West Africa, accounting for a significant proportion of global malaria cases. Malaria transmission is widespread throughout the country, with regional variations in prevalence and burden. Understanding these variations and targeting interventions to specific regions, particularly the higher burden areas, is essential in reducing the impact of malaria in Nigeria.

Ghana is another West African country heavily affected by malaria, with high transmission rates observed in many regions (WHO, 2020). This indicates the significant burden of malaria in the country and the need for robust control measures. Malaria accounts for a substantial proportion of outpatient visits and hospital admissions in Ghana, reflecting the impact of the disease on the healthcare system (WHO, 2020).

Regional variations within Ghana contribute to different malaria prevalence rates. Generally, the northern regions of Ghana experience higher malaria prevalence compared to the southern regions (Noland et al., 2020). Factors such as climate, ecological conditions, and socioeconomic factors contribute to these regional disparities. The northern regions, with their warmer temperatures and more suitable breeding conditions for mosquitoes, face greater challenges in controlling malaria transmission.

Recognizing these regional variations is crucial for implementing targeted interventions to address the malaria burden in Ghana effectively. Efforts should be focused on the higher burden areas, particularly in the northern regions. These interventions may include the distribution of insecticide-treated bed nets, access to prompt diagnosis and effective treatment, and implementation of vector control strategies.

To combat malaria in Ghana, a comprehensive approach is needed that considers the unique challenges and characteristics of each region. Collaboration between the government, healthcare institutions, non-governmental organizations, and local communities is essential for the successful implementation and sustainability of malaria control programs.

In conclusion, Ghana is heavily affected by malaria, with high transmission rates observed in many regions. Malaria accounts for a significant proportion of outpatient visits and hospital admissions in the country. Regional variations in malaria prevalence exist, with higher prevalence typically found in the northern regions compared to the southern regions. Understanding these variations and implementing targeted interventions are crucial in reducing the malaria burden in Ghana.

2.2.3 Burkina Faso:

Burkina Faso experiences a high malaria burden, with transmission occurring throughout the year (WHO, 2020). This indicates that the population is at continuous risk of malaria infection, emphasizing the urgent need for effective control measures. Malaria is a leading cause of morbidity and mortality in Burkina Faso, particularly among children under the age of five (WHO, 2020). The vulnerability of this age group highlights the importance of targeted interventions to protect their health and well-being.

Regional variations within Burkina Faso contribute to different malaria prevalence rates. Generally, the southern regions of Burkina Faso have higher malaria prevalence compared to the northern regions (Noland et al., 2020). Factors such as climate, ecological conditions, and socioeconomic factors contribute to these regional disparities. The southern regions, with their warmer temperatures and higher humidity, provide suitable conditions for malaria transmission.

Recognizing these regional variations is essential for implementing targeted interventions to effectively address the malaria burden in Burkina Faso. Efforts should be focused on the higher prevalence areas, particularly in the southern regions. These interventions may include the distribution of insecticide-treated bed nets, access to prompt diagnosis and effective treatment, and implementation of vector control strategies.

A comprehensive approach is needed to combat malaria in Burkina Faso, considering the unique challenges and characteristics of each region. Collaboration between the government, healthcare institutions, non-governmental organizations, and local communities is crucial for the successful implementation and sustainability of malaria control programs.

Mali is significantly affected by malaria, experiencing high transmission rates and a substantial malaria burden (WHO, 2020). This highlights the urgent need for effective control measures to combat the disease in the country. Malaria is a leading cause of illness and death in Mali, particularly among children under the age of five and pregnant women (WHO, 2020). These vulnerable populations require targeted interventions to reduce the morbidity and mortality associated with malaria.

Regional variations within Mali contribute to different malaria prevalence rates. Generally, the southern regions of Mali have higher malaria prevalence compared to the northern regions (Noland et al., 2020). Factors such as climate, ecological conditions, and socioeconomic factors influence these regional disparities. The southern regions, characterized by higher temperatures and more favorable breeding conditions for mosquitoes, are more susceptible to malaria transmission.

Recognizing these regional variations is crucial for implementing targeted interventions to effectively address the malaria burden in Mali. Efforts should be focused on the higher prevalence areas, particularly in the southern regions. These interventions may include the distribution of insecticide-treated bed nets, access to prompt diagnosis and effective treatment, and implementation of vector control strategies.

A comprehensive approach is necessary to combat malaria in Mali, taking into account the unique challenges and characteristics of each region. Collaboration between the government, healthcare institutions, non-governmental organizations, and local communities is crucial for the successful implementation and sustainability of malaria control programs.

It is important to note that while the above countries are highlighted as being heavily affected by malaria, several other West

THE IMPACT OF MALARIA ON THE SOCIAL-ECONOMIC DEVELOPMENT OF WEST AFRICA

African countries, including Benin, Ivory Coast, Senegal, and Sierra Leone, also experience a significant malaria burden and face challenges in malaria control and prevention efforts.

Understanding the most affected countries and regions within West Africa helps prioritize resources, interventions, and policy measures to combat malaria effectively in these areas.

Table 2: information on the most affected countries and regions in West Africa:

Country	Malaria Burden	Regional Variations
Nigeria	Accounts for 25% of global malaria cases; widespread transmission throughout the country (WHO)	Higher prevalence and burden in northern regions (Noland et al., 2020)
Ghana	High transmission rates observed in many regions; significant impact on healthcare system (WHO)	Higher prevalence in northern regions compared to southern regions (Noland et al., 2020)
Burkina Faso	High malaria burden; year-round transmission; leading cause of morbidity and mortality (WHO)	Higher prevalence in southern regions compared to northern regions (Noland et al., 2020)
Mali	High transmission rates; substantial malaria burden; significant impact on vulnerable populations (WHO)	Higher prevalence in southern regions compared to northern regions (Noland et al., 2020)

The table provides a summary of the malaria burden in each country and highlights the regional variations in malaria prevalence.

2.3 Examination of the factors contributing to the high malaria transmission rates in West Africa

Several factors contribute to the high malaria transmission rates observed in West Africa. Understanding these factors is crucial for implementing effective control and prevention strategies.

2.3.1 Climate and ecology:

West Africa's climate plays a crucial role in facilitating malaria transmission, as highlighted by Tusting et al. (2020). The region's high temperatures and rainfall create favorable conditions for the survival and reproduction of malaria vectors, primarily mosquitoes. These climatic factors contribute to the proliferation of mosquito populations, increasing the risk of malaria transmission.

The diverse ecosystems found in West Africa, including forests, savannahs, and wetlands, also play a significant role in malaria transmission (Tusting et al., 2020). These ecosystems provide suitable breeding grounds for malaria-carrying mosquitoes. Forested areas, for instance, often have high mosquito densities due to the presence of shaded and humid environments, creating ideal conditions for mosquito breeding.

Environmental changes, such as deforestation and urbanization, can further impact malaria transmission dynamics in West Africa (Bogoch et al., 2020). Deforestation alters the ecological balance, disrupting natural habitats and potentially increasing human-mosquito contact. Urbanization, with its associated population density and inadequate infrastructure, can create conditions conducive to mosquito breeding and facilitate the spread of malaria in urban areas.

Understanding the link between climate, ecology, and malaria transmission is crucial for designing effective control strategies. Implementing vector control measures, such as insecticide-treated bed nets, indoor residual spraying, and larval source management, can help reduce mosquito populations and interrupt malaria transmission. Additionally, monitoring and adapting to environmental changes, such as deforestation and urbanization, are essential for mitigating the impact on malaria transmission dynamics.

2.3.2 Vector species and behavior:

In West Africa, Anopheles mosquitoes, specifically Anopheles gambiae and Anopheles funestus, play a crucial role as primary malaria vectors, as identified by Bhatt et al. (2015). These mosquito species are responsible for the majority of malaria transmission in the region.

Anopheles gambiae and Anopheles funestus are known for their high biting rates, meaning they have a greater likelihood of biting humans and transmitting the malaria parasite (Bhatt et al., 2015). These mosquito species exhibit strong anthropophilic tendencies, displaying a preference for feeding on human blood. This behavior increases the risk of malaria transmission as mosquitoes come into contact with infected individuals and subsequently transmit the parasites to other individuals they subsequently bite.

Moreover, these mosquito species have efficient transmission capabilities, meaning they can effectively acquire, sustain, and transmit the malaria parasite (Bhatt et al., 2015). This efficiency contributes to the persistence and endemicity of malaria in West Africa.

A significant challenge in malaria control efforts is the emergence of vector resistance to insecticides. Hemingway et al. (2020) highlight that mosquitoes in West Africa have developed resistance to commonly used insecticides, making it more difficult to control mosquito populations and interrupt malaria transmission. This resistance can be attributed to several factors, including the extensive use of insecticides in agricultural practices and public health interventions. Efforts are underway to develop and deploy alternative vector control strategies to overcome insecticide resistance.

Understanding the behavior and characteristics of Anopheles mosquitoes, as well as their resistance to insecticides, is crucial for implementing effective vector control measures. Integrated vector management approaches, including the use of insecticide-treated bed nets, indoor residual spraying, larval source management, and the development of novel insecticides, can help overcome the challenges posed by mosquito vectors and reduce malaria transmission.

Chapter 3. Socio-economic factors and population movements:

P overty, inadequate housing, and limited access to healthcare are significant contributing factors to increased malaria vulnerability and transmission in West Africa, as highlighted by Bogoch et al. (2020). These socio-economic challenges create conditions that facilitate the proliferation of malaria-carrying mosquitoes and hinder effective prevention and control measures. Below are significant factors to consider:

3.1.1 The Interplay of Poverty and Malaria in West Africa

Poverty exacerbates the risk of malaria in West Africa, as impoverished communities often lack resources for malaria prevention and treatment. Limited access to insecticide-treated bed nets, effective antimalarial drugs, and healthcare services hinders the ability to protect individuals from malaria infection and provide timely treatment.

3.1.1.1 Housing Conditions and Malaria Risk

INADEQUATE HOUSING conditions, such as inadequate sanitation, improper drainage systems, and insufficient housing structures, create favorable environments for mosquito breeding and increase human-mosquito contact. Stagnant water, often found in and around poorly constructed dwellings, serves as breeding grounds for malaria vectors.

3.1.1.2 Access to Healthcare Services and the Malaria Burden in West Africa:

LIMITED ACCESS TO HEALTHCARE services further exacerbates the malaria burden in West Africa. Insufficient healthcare infrastructure, including a shortage of healthcare facilities, trained healthcare workers, and diagnostic tools, hampers prompt diagnosis and effective treatment. This results in delayed or inadequate management of malaria cases, leading to increased morbidity and mortality.

3.1.1.3 Population movement and migration

POPULATION MOVEMENTS, including migration and displacement, contribute to the introduction and spread of malaria in new areas. Cohen et al. (2017) emphasize that the movement of individuals from high transmission areas to low transmission areas can introduce malaria parasites into previously unaffected regions. Additionally, population displacement due to conflicts or natural disasters can lead to overcrowding, inadequate housing conditions, and disrupted healthcare systems, further increasing malaria vulnerability and transmission.

Addressing the socio-economic determinants of malaria vulnerability is crucial for effective malaria control in West Africa. Efforts should focus on poverty alleviation, improving housing conditions, and strengthening healthcare systems. This includes providing access to affordable and quality healthcare services, ensuring the availability of insecticide-treated bed nets, implementing vector control strategies, and promoting community engagement and education on malaria prevention and treatment.

3.1.2 Lack of access to prevention and control interventions:

The lack of access to prevention and control interventions plays a significant role in the high malaria transmission rates in West Africa, as highlighted by Bogoch et al. (2020). Several factors contribute to this issue:

3.1.2.1 Challenges in the Availability and Utilization of Malaria Prevention Measures and Treatments in West Africa

LIMITED AVAILABILITY and utilization of insecticide-treated bed nets, indoor residual spraying (IRS), and effective antimalarial treatments contribute to the persistence of malaria transmission. Insecticide-treated bed nets are a crucial preventive measure, but their availability and utilization remain low in some areas. Similarly, indoor residual spraying, which involves applying insecticides to the interior walls of houses, is an effective vector control strategy but may face challenges in implementation and coverage. Additionally, the availability and accessibility of effective antimalarial treatments can be limited in certain regions, leading to inadequate management of malaria cases.

3.1.2.2 Impediments to Effective Malaria Control: Challenges in Healthcare Infrastructure and Delivery Systems

CHALLENGES IN HEALTHCARE infrastructure and delivery systems hinder the effective implementation of malaria control measures. Insufficient healthcare facilities, shortage of trained healthcare workers, and limited diagnostic tools hamper prompt diagnosis and effective treatment of malaria cases. Inadequate laboratory capacity for malaria diagnosis, especially in remote areas, can result in delayed or inaccurate diagnoses, leading to suboptimal management of malaria cases.

Addressing the lack of access to prevention and control interventions requires comprehensive efforts. This includes strengthening healthcare infrastructure, improving supply chain management to ensure the availability of essential malaria interventions, and enhancing healthcare delivery systems. Increasing accessibility and affordability of insecticide-treated bed nets and antimalarial treatments, as well as improving coverage of IRS campaigns, are vital for reducing malaria transmission rates.

Community engagement and education are also crucial in promoting the utilization of prevention and control interventions. Public awareness campaigns can enhance knowledge about malaria prevention and treatment, improving community participation and uptake of interventions.

3.1.3 Drug resistance:

The emergence and spread of antimalarial drug resistance, particularly to artemisinin-based combination therapies (ACTs), pose a significant threat to malaria control efforts in West Africa, as highlighted by Takala-Harrison et al. (2013). Artemisinin, a key component of ACTs, is an effective and widely used antimalarial drug. However, the development of resistance to artemisinin and its partner drugs undermines the efficacy of these treatments.

Drug-resistant malaria parasites have the ability to survive and continue transmission, posing challenges to treatment effectiveness and potentially increasing malaria transmission rates. When parasites become resistant to ACTs, they can persist in infected individuals despite treatment, leading to prolonged illness and increased risk of transmission to mosquitoes.

The spread of drug-resistant malaria parasites is a complex process influenced by several factors, including genetic mutations in the parasites and selective pressure from the use of antimalarial drugs. Resistance can emerge and spread rapidly, particularly in areas with intense malaria transmission and high drug usage.

Dealing with drug resistance requires a multi-faceted approach. Strategies include monitoring the efficacy of antimalarial drugs through regular surveillance, implementing appropriate treatment protocols based on drug resistance patterns, and promoting rational drug use to minimize the development and spread of resistance. Combination therapies and novel antimalarial drugs are being developed and tested to overcome resistance and provide effective treatment options.

Additionally, efforts to prevent malaria transmission through vector control interventions, such as insecticide-treated bed nets and indoor residual spraying, can reduce the overall burden of malaria and limit the spread of drug-resistant parasites.

These factors interact in complex ways, leading to sustained malaria transmission in West Africa. Addressing these factors through a comprehensive approach, including vector control, access to prevention measures, healthcare infrastructure improvements, and research on drug resistance, is essential to reduce malaria transmission rates in the region.

Chapter 4. Health Impact of Malaria in West Africa

43

4.1 Health consequences of malaria infection

Malaria infection can have a wide range of health consequences, particularly in areas with high transmission rates like West Africa. The following discussion highlights the key health consequences of malaria, supported by relevant in-text citations:

4.1.1 Fever and flu-like symptoms:

Malaria typically presents with symptoms that resemble a severe flu-like illness, including high fever, chills, headache, and body aches (WHO, 2020). These symptoms can be debilitating and have a significant impact on an individual's daily activities and productivity.

The high fever associated with malaria can cause fatigue, weakness, and loss of appetite, making it challenging for individuals to perform their regular tasks. The chills and body aches can lead to discomfort and difficulty in movement, further hindering productivity.

The headache associated with malaria can be severe and persistent, affecting concentration and cognitive function. This can make it difficult for individuals to focus on work or academic activities, reducing productivity.

Moreover, malaria symptoms can occur in cycles, with periodic episodes of fever and illness. This recurrent pattern can lead to prolonged periods of illness and recovery, resulting in significant time off from work or school.

In addition to the physical symptoms, malaria can also have psychological and emotional effects. The illness can cause anxiety, stress, and worry, which can further impact an individual's well-being and ability to perform daily activities effectively.

Early diagnosis and prompt treatment of malaria are crucial to alleviate symptoms, prevent complications, and minimize the impact on productivity. Access to healthcare services, accurate diagnostic tools, and effective antimalarial treatments are essential in managing malaria cases and reducing the burden of the disease.

In certain cases, malaria can progress to severe forms that pose significant risks to health and life. Severe malaria can manifest as severe anemia, cerebral malaria (infection of the brain), acute respiratory distress syndrome (ARDS), and multi-organ failure (WHO, 2020).

Severe anemia occurs when malaria parasites destroy red blood cells at an accelerated rate, leading to a significant decrease in hemoglobin levels. This can result in fatigue, weakness, organ dysfunction, and, in severe cases, require blood transfusions for treatment.

Cerebral malaria is a severe complication characterized by the infection of the brain by malaria parasites. It can lead to coma, seizures, neurological deficits, and long-term cognitive impairments if not promptly treated.

Acute respiratory distress syndrome (ARDS) can occur as a result of the severe inflammation triggered by malaria infection. It causes a rapid onset of respiratory failure, often requiring mechanical ventilation and intensive care management.

Multi-organ failure can arise from the widespread impact of malaria parasites on various organ systems, including the liver, kidneys, and cardiovascular system. It can lead to organ dysfunction and failure, significantly increasing the risk of mortality.

Severe malaria poses a high risk of mortality, particularly among vulnerable populations such as children under the age of five and pregnant women (WHO, 2020). These individuals may have compromised immune systems and reduced physiological reserves, making them more susceptible to severe complications.

Timely diagnosis and prompt treatment are critical in preventing the progression to severe malaria and reducing the associated mortality. Access to quality healthcare, early recognition of symptoms, and appropriate antimalarial therapies are essential for managing severe malaria cases.

4.1.3 Anemia:

Malaria is indeed a leading cause of anemia in endemic regions. The malaria parasite destroys red blood cells, leading to a decrease in the number of circulating red blood cells and hemoglobin levels in the body (WHO, 2020). This destruction of red blood cells contributes to the development of anemia.

Anemia, characterized by a lower than normal level of hemoglobin in the blood, can have significant impacts on individuals. The symptoms of anemia include fatigue, weakness, and a decreased ability to perform physical activities. These symptoms can have a substantial impact on the daily lives and productivity of individuals affected by malaria-related anemia.

In children, anemia resulting from malaria can have long-term consequences for cognitive development. Chronic anemia during childhood can impair cognitive function, including memory, attention, and learning abilities. This can hinder educational attainment and limit future opportunities for affected children.

Pregnant women are particularly vulnerable to malaria-related anemia. Anemia during pregnancy increases the risk of complications such as maternal mortality, premature birth, low birth weight, and impaired fetal development. It is crucial to address malaria and prevent anemia in pregnant women to ensure optimal health outcomes for both the mother and the child.

Preventing and treating malaria is key to reducing the burden of malaria-related anemia. Prompt diagnosis and effective treatment of malaria cases can help prevent further destruction of red blood cells and mitigate the development of anemia. Additionally, strategies to prevent malaria transmission, such as the use of insecticide-treated bed nets, indoor residual spraying, and intermittent preventive treatment in pregnant women, can contribute to reducing the incidence of malaria-related anemia.

THE IMPACT OF MALARIA ON THE SOCIAL-ECONOMIC DEVELOPMENT OF WEST AFRICA

In conclusion, malaria is a leading cause of anemia in endemic regions. The destruction of red blood cells by the malaria parasite contributes to the development of anemia. Anemia resulting from malaria can lead to fatigue, weakness, impaired cognitive development in children, and complications during pregnancy. Preventing and treating malaria is crucial in reducing the burden of malaria-related anemia and improving the overall health and well-being of affected individuals.

4.1.4 Pregnancy-related complications:

Pregnant women face increased vulnerability to malaria infection, with serious consequences for both the mother and the child. Malaria infection during pregnancy is associated with various complications, as highlighted by the World Health Organization (WHO, 2020).

One of the significant risks of malaria in pregnancy is maternal anemia, which can result from the destruction of red blood cells by the malaria parasite. Maternal anemia can lead to fatigue, weakness, and reduced oxygen-carrying capacity, affecting the overall health and well-being of the mother.

Malaria in pregnancy is also linked to adverse birth outcomes, including low birth weight and preterm delivery. The infection can impair the growth and development of the fetus, resulting in infants with lower birth weights. Low birth weight is associated with an increased risk of infant mortality, as well as developmental delays and long-term health issues.

Furthermore, malaria in pregnancy increases the risk of maternal and neonatal mortality. Severe cases of malaria can lead to complications such as organ failure, which can be life-threatening for both the mother and the baby.

The long-term effects of malaria in pregnancy extend beyond childbirth. Desai et al. (2018) highlight that malaria infection during pregnancy can have lasting impacts on the health and development of both the mother and the child. These effects can include cognitive impairments, increased susceptibility to infections, and compromised immune function.

Preventing malaria in pregnancy is crucial for protecting the health of both the mother and the child. Interventions such as intermittent preventive treatment during pregnancy (IPTp) with antimalarial drugs and the use of insecticide-treated bed nets are recommended to reduce the risk of malaria infection and its associated complications.

Ensuring access to quality antenatal care, including regular screening for malaria, prompt diagnosis, and effective treatment, is vital for the well-being of pregnant women. Additionally, education and awareness programs targeting pregnant women and healthcare providers can help promote preventive measures and timely intervention.

4.1.5 Impaired cognitive development:

Malaria infections, particularly in young children, can have detrimental effects on cognitive development, as highlighted by Fernando et al. (2016). The impact of malaria on cognitive function is particularly significant when infections occur during critical periods of brain development.

Recurrent episodes of malaria can interrupt normal brain development, leading to neurocognitive impairments. Malaria parasites can cause inflammation and damage to brain tissue, affecting neural pathways and cognitive functions. The interruption of normal brain development can result in difficulties with learning, memory, attention, and other cognitive processes.

The long-term consequences of impaired cognitive development can have a significant impact on academic performance and educational attainment. Children affected by malaria-related cognitive impairments may struggle to keep up with their peers in school and face challenges in acquiring and retaining knowledge. This can lead to lower educational achievements and limited future opportunities.

Furthermore, the cognitive impairments resulting from malaria infections can persist into adulthood and have implications for overall well-being and quality of life. Individuals may experience difficulties in employment, social relationships, and daily functioning due to their cognitive limitations.

Preventing and treating malaria in children is crucial for mitigating the impact on cognitive development. Strategies such as the use of insecticide-treated bed nets, indoor residual spraying, and prompt diagnosis and treatment of malaria cases are essential for reducing the frequency and severity of infections.

Early childhood interventions, including nutritional support, stimulation programs, and access to quality education, can help mitigate the effects of impaired cognitive development and support affected children in reaching their full potential.

In conclusion, malaria infections, particularly in young children, can lead to neurocognitive impairments that affect learning abilities, school performance, and long-term cognitive development. Recurrent episodes of malaria during critical periods of brain development can have lasting effects on cognitive function. Preventing and treating malaria in children is crucial for mitigating the impact on cognitive development and ensuring optimal educational outcomes and overall well-being.

4.1.6 Impact on overall health and well-being:

$\mathbf{M}$alaria can indeed have a significant impact on overall health and well-being, contributing to a cycle of poverty and poor health. Littrell et al. (2013) highlight several aspects of this impact.

Malaria infections can lead to frequent episodes of illness and hospitalizations, causing a substantial burden on affected individuals. The debilitating symptoms, such as high fever, chills, and fatigue, can leave individuals unable to perform their daily activities and work. This can result in lost productivity and income, further exacerbating the cycle of poverty.

The recovery period from malaria infections can be lengthy, depending on the severity of the disease and the individual's overall health. The need for rest and recuperation can disrupt daily routines and hinder individuals' ability to engage in productive activities, including work and education.

The economic burden of malaria extends beyond the direct costs of treatment. The cost of healthcare services, diagnostic tests, medications, and transportation to healthcare facilities can impose a financial strain on affected individuals and their families. These healthcare expenditures can lead to further impoverishment and limit access to other essential goods and services.

Moreover, malaria can have indirect costs on households and communities. When individuals are unable to work due to illness or caretaking responsibilities, it can strain household resources and reduce income-generating opportunities. This can perpetuate the cycle of poverty and hinder overall socio-economic development.

Addressing the impact of malaria on overall health and well-being requires a comprehensive approach. It involves not only effective prevention and treatment of malaria but also addressing the underlying determinants of poverty and improving access to quality healthcare and social support systems.

Efforts to control and eliminate malaria should be integrated into broader health and development strategies, addressing poverty, improving education, and strengthening healthcare systems. This includes increasing access to malaria prevention measures, such as insecticide-treated bed nets and indoor residual spraying, as well as improving the availability and affordability of antimalarial treatments.

It is important to note that effective treatment and prevention measures can significantly reduce the health consequences of malaria. Prompt diagnosis, access to appropriate antimalarial medications, and preventive interventions such as insecticide-treated bed nets and indoor residual spraying play crucial roles in mitigating the health impacts of malaria.

Table 3: Health consequences of malaria infection:

Health Consequences	Description
Fever and flu-like symptoms	Malaria presents with symptoms similar to a severe flu-like illness, including high fever, chills, headache, and body aches.
Severe malaria	In severe cases, malaria can lead to complications such as severe anemia, cerebral malaria, acute respiratory distress syndrome, and multi-organ failure.
Anemia	Malaria contributes to the development of anemia, resulting in fatigue, weakness, and cognitive impairments.
Pregnancy-related complications	Malaria in pregnancy increases the risk of maternal anemia, low birth weight, preterm delivery, and maternal and neonatal mortality.
Impaired cognitive development	Malaria infections, especially in children, can lead to cognitive impairments, affecting learning abilities and academic performance.
Impact on overall health and well-being	Malaria can cause frequent illness, hospitalizations, economic burden, and hinder socio-economic development.

These health consequences highlight the importance of effective prevention, early diagnosis, and prompt treatment to mitigate the impact of malaria on individuals' well-being.

4.2 Impact on mortality rates, particularly among children and pregnant women

Malaria has a significant impact on mortality rates, particularly among children under five and pregnant women in malaria-endemic regions like West Africa. The following discussion explores the mortality burden of malaria in these vulnerable populations:

Malaria poses a significant threat to the health and well-being of children under five years old, particularly in malaria-endemic regions. The World Health Organization (WHO, 2020) emphasizes the following points:

Malaria is a leading cause of death among children under five, especially in areas where malaria transmission is high. In sub-Saharan Africa, which includes West Africa, approximately 260,000 child deaths are attributed to malaria each year.

Severe malaria and its associated complications play a crucial role in the high mortality rates among young children. Severe forms of malaria, such as severe anemia and cerebral malaria, can have life-threatening consequences.

Severe anemia, a condition characterized by a significant decrease in red blood cells and hemoglobin levels, can lead to organ dysfunction and impaired oxygen transport. It is a common complication of malaria in young children and contributes to the increased mortality rates.

Cerebral malaria, which occurs when the malaria parasite affects the brain, can lead to coma, seizures, and neurological damage. This severe form of malaria has a high mortality rate, particularly among young children.

The vulnerability of young children to malaria-related complications is due to several factors, including their immature immune systems and limited access to appropriate healthcare services.

The underdeveloped immune systems of young children make them more susceptible to severe malaria and its complications.

Preventing and treating malaria in children under five is crucial in reducing child mortality rates. Strategies such as the use of insecticide-treated bed nets, indoor residual spraying, prompt diagnosis, and effective treatment are vital for protecting young children from malaria infection and its severe consequences.

4.2.1 Pregnant women:

Pregnant women face an elevated risk of severe malaria and related complications, which significantly increases mortality rates, as emphasized by the World Health Organization (WHO, 2020).

Malaria in pregnancy is a significant contributor to maternal mortality, particularly in sub-Saharan Africa, including West Africa. It is estimated that approximately 10,000 maternal deaths occur annually in this region due to malaria.

Complications associated with malaria infections during pregnancy contribute to the mortality burden among pregnant women. Severe anemia, a condition characterized by a significant decrease in red blood cells and hemoglobin levels, can occur as a result of malaria and lead to organ dysfunction. Placental malaria, the presence of malaria parasites in the placenta, can cause adverse outcomes such as fetal growth restriction, low birth weight, and maternal complications. Malaria infections during pregnancy can also increase the risk of preterm birth, which carries its own risks for both the mother and the baby.

The immune changes that occur during pregnancy make women more susceptible to severe malaria and its complications. The physiological adaptations of pregnancy, including changes in the immune response and increased blood volume, can provide favorable conditions for malaria parasites to replicate and cause more severe disease.

Preventing and managing malaria in pregnancy is essential for reducing maternal mortality rates. Interventions such as intermittent preventive treatment in pregnancy (IPTp) with antimalarial drugs and the use of insecticide-treated bed nets are recommended to protect pregnant women from malaria infections and related complications.

Early and regular antenatal care, including prompt diagnosis and effective treatment of malaria cases, is crucial in minimizing the impact of malaria on pregnant women. Adequate nutrition, iron and folic acid supplementation, and access to skilled delivery care further contribute to reducing maternal mortality associated with malaria.

4.2.2 Impact of malaria control interventions:

The implementation of effective malaria control interventions has had a significant impact on reducing mortality rates among children and pregnant women, as highlighted by O'Meara et al. (2010).

The use of insecticide-treated bed nets (ITNs) is a key strategy in preventing malaria transmission. ITNs create a physical barrier against mosquito bites and can reduce malaria-related morbidity and mortality. Studies have demonstrated that the widespread use of ITNs can significantly reduce the risk of malaria infection and related complications, particularly among vulnerable populations such as children and pregnant women.

Antimalarial medications, such as artemisinin-based combination therapies (ACTs), are crucial for the effective treatment of malaria cases. Timely and appropriate treatment with ACTs can prevent the progression of uncomplicated malaria to severe forms, reducing the risk of mortality. Access to these antimalarial medications has been associated with a significant reduction in malaria-related deaths, particularly among children and pregnant women.

The increased coverage and access to malaria control interventions have led to substantial declines in malaria-related mortality in several endemic countries. The scale-up of interventions such as ITNs and ACTs has been associated with significant reductions in the burden of malaria, including a decline in mortality rates among the most vulnerable populations.

It is important to note that the success of malaria control interventions depends on various factors, including the coverage and quality of interventions, community engagement, and health system strengthening. Sustained efforts to ensure universal access to these interventions and their effective implementation are crucial for achieving further reductions in malaria-related mortality.

62

4.2.3 Challenges in reducing mortality rates:

Reducing malaria-related mortality rates among vulnerable populations faces several challenges, as highlighted by Gething et al. (2016).

Access to healthcare facilities is a significant challenge in many malaria-endemic regions, particularly in remote and underserved areas. Limited availability of healthcare facilities and long distances to reach them can hinder timely access to diagnosis and treatment. This can result in delays in receiving appropriate care, allowing the infection to progress to severe forms and increasing the risk of mortality.

Delays in seeking appropriate treatment also contribute to the mortality burden. Lack of awareness about malaria symptoms, cultural beliefs, and financial constraints can prevent individuals from seeking healthcare promptly. Delayed treatment can lead to the worsening of malaria symptoms and the development of severe complications, increasing the likelihood of mortality.

The emergence and spread of drug resistance pose a considerable challenge in malaria control efforts. Resistance to antimalarial drugs, particularly to artemisinin-based combination therapies (ACTs), can reduce treatment effectiveness and contribute to treatment failures. Limited availability of alternative effective antimalarial drugs further exacerbates the challenge of reducing mortality rates.

Delays in diagnosis also contribute to the mortality burden. Rapid and accurate diagnosis is crucial for timely initiation of appropriate treatment. However, limited access to diagnostic tools and trained healthcare providers in some settings can lead to delays in diagnosing malaria cases, particularly in remote areas.

Insufficient resources, including financial resources and healthcare infrastructure, pose additional challenges. Limited funding for malaria control programs can hinder the scale-up of interventions and the delivery of essential healthcare services. Inadequate healthcare infrastructure, including laboratories and healthcare personnel, can limit the capacity to diagnose and treat malaria cases effectively.

Addressing these challenges requires comprehensive approaches. Strengthening healthcare systems, improving access to quality healthcare services, and enhancing community engagement and education are essential. Efforts to combat drug resistance and ensure the availability of effective antimalarial drugs are critical. Additionally, investments in research and innovation to develop new tools and strategies for malaria control are crucial for reducing mortality rates.

Efforts to reduce malaria-related mortality rates among children and pregnant women in West Africa require a comprehensive approach that includes preventive measures, early diagnosis, prompt treatment, and improved access to healthcare services. Sustained investment in malaria control programs and research to develop new interventions and combat drug resistance is crucial to further reduce mortality rates in these vulnerable populations.

4.3 Analysis of the long-term effects of repeated malaria infections on individuals' health and well-being

Repeated malaria infections, particularly in malaria-endemic regions like West Africa, can have long-term effects on individuals' health and well-being. The following analysis explores the impact of repeated malaria infections on various aspects of individuals' health, supported by relevant information and studies:

4.3.1 Cognitive development and education:

Repeated episodes of malaria during childhood can have long-term consequences on neurocognitive development, which can impact learning abilities and educational attainment, as highlighted by Fernando et al. (2016).

Malaria-related cognitive impairments can contribute to lower academic performance and educational outcomes, particularly in malaria-endemic areas. The cognitive impairments resulting from malaria infections, such as difficulties with attention, memory, and information processing, can hinder children's ability to acquire and retain knowledge, negatively affecting their learning abilities. This can lead to lower academic achievements and limited educational opportunities.

The long-term effects of malaria on cognitive development can have profound implications for individuals' potential for personal and socio-economic advancement. Impaired cognitive abilities can limit individuals' capacity to pursue higher education, gain employment in certain fields, and engage in complex cognitive tasks required for socio-economic success. These long-term effects can perpetuate cycles of poverty and hinder overall socio-economic development in endemic areas.

It is important to recognize the potential impact of malaria on cognitive development and implement appropriate interventions. Strategies such as early diagnosis and prompt treatment of malaria cases, access to quality education, nutritional support, and psychosocial interventions can help mitigate the cognitive impairments associated with repeated episodes of malaria. Additionally, investment in research and innovation to develop effective interventions for preventing and treating malaria in children is essential for reducing the long-term cognitive consequences.

4.3.2 Anemia and nutritional status:

Repeated malaria infections can indeed contribute to chronic anemia, as highlighted by the World Health Organization (WHO, 2020). Malaria-associated anemia occurs when the malaria parasite destroys red blood cells, leading to a decrease in hemoglobin levels.

Chronic anemia resulting from malaria can have significant consequences on individuals' health and well-being. The symptoms of anemia, including fatigue, weakness, and shortness of breath, can limit individuals' physical activities and reduce their overall productivity. These symptoms can have a detrimental impact on individuals' quality of life and hinder their ability to engage in daily activities and work effectively.

Moreover, the burden of anemia resulting from malaria can further exacerbate the problem of malnutrition. Anemia can impair individuals' appetite and their body's ability to absorb and utilize nutrients effectively. This can lead to a vicious cycle where malnutrition contributes to anemia, which, in turn, worsens the state of malnutrition. The combined effects of anemia and malnutrition can have profound consequences on overall health, growth, and development, particularly among children.

In addition to the physical effects, anemia resulting from malaria can also impact cognitive development. Chronic anemia can impair cognitive function, affecting learning abilities and school performance, as well as contributing to reduced attention span and decreased memory retention.

Addressing the burden of anemia resulting from malaria requires a multifaceted approach. This includes effective prevention and treatment of malaria infections, access to appropriate antimalarial medications, and nutritional interventions to address underlying malnutrition. Additionally, improving overall healthcare infrastructure, including access to diagnostic tools and healthcare providers, is crucial for timely diagnosis and management of malaria-related anemia.

4.3.3 Impact on economic productivity:

Frequent episodes of malaria can indeed have a significant impact on economic productivity, as highlighted by Littrell et al. (2013).

Malaria-related illnesses can result in reduced productivity among affected individuals. The symptoms of malaria, such as high fever, fatigue, and body aches, can significantly impair individuals' ability to carry out their regular work activities. This can lead to decreased productivity and a loss of income for both the affected individuals and their employers.

Furthermore, the need for treatment and recovery periods following malaria infections can result in work absenteeism. Individuals may need to take time off from work to seek medical care, rest, and recuperate. This can further contribute to economic losses, particularly for those in informal or daily wage employment who may not have access to sick leave or other forms of employment protection.

The economic impact of malaria extends beyond the individual level and affects societies as a whole. High malaria prevalence in communities can lead to a significant loss of productivity at the societal level. The cumulative effect of reduced productivity and work absenteeism among individuals can hinder overall economic development and perpetuate cycles of poverty.

In addition to the direct impact on productivity, malaria-related illnesses and treatment costs can impose a financial burden on affected individuals and their families. Expenses related to healthcare services, diagnostic tests, medications, and transportation to healthcare facilities can strain household resources and contribute to economic hardship. This financial burden can perpetuate the cycle of poverty and limit access to other essential goods and services.

Addressing the impact of malaria on economic productivity requires comprehensive interventions. Effective malaria prevention measures, such as the use of insecticide-treated bed nets and indoor residual spraying, can reduce the incidence of malaria and its associated economic burden. Access to prompt and affordable diagnosis and treatment of malaria cases is crucial to minimize the duration and severity of illness and reduce the economic impact. Additionally, investments in health systems strengthening and poverty alleviation strategies can contribute to sustainable improvements in economic productivity in malaria-endemic regions.

4.3.4 Implications for pregnancy outcomes:

Repeated malaria infections in pregnant women can indeed increase the risk of adverse pregnancy outcomes, as highlighted by the World Health Organization (WHO, 2020).

Malaria infections during pregnancy can lead to a higher likelihood of low birth weight, which is defined as a birth weight of less than 2,500 grams. Low birth weight is associated with an increased risk of neonatal mortality and long-term health complications for the infant.

Preterm delivery, the birth of a baby before completing 37 weeks of gestation, is also more likely to occur in pregnant women with malaria infections. Preterm babies may face challenges related to their development and may require specialized care in neonatal units.

Malaria in pregnancy can also contribute to maternal complications. Severe anemia, a condition characterized by a significant decrease in red blood cells and hemoglobin levels, is a common complication of malaria during pregnancy. Severe anemia can lead to maternal fatigue, weakness, and increased vulnerability to other infections.

The presence of malaria parasites in the placenta, known as placental malaria, is another complication that can occur during pregnancy. Placental malaria can lead to impaired nutrient and oxygen exchange between the mother and the fetus, potentially affecting the growth and development of the baby.

These adverse pregnancy outcomes resulting from malaria infections can have long-term consequences for both the mother and the child. Low birth weight is associated with increased risks of infant mortality, stunted growth, and impaired cognitive and physical development. Preterm birth can lead to developmental delays and health issues for the baby. Maternal complications, such as severe anemia, can impact the mother's well-being and increase the risk of maternal mortality.

THE IMPACT OF MALARIA ON THE SOCIAL-ECONOMIC DEVELOPMENT OF WEST AFRICA

Preventing and managing malaria infections during pregnancy is crucial for reducing the risk of adverse pregnancy outcomes. Interventions such as intermittent preventive treatment in pregnancy (IPTp) with antimalarial drugs, the use of insecticide-treated bed nets, and access to quality antenatal care can help protect pregnant women from malaria and minimize the associated risks. Timely diagnosis and appropriate treatment of malaria cases in pregnant women are also essential.

4.3.5 Vulnerability to other infections and diseases:

Malaria can weaken the immune system, making individuals more susceptible to other infections and diseases. (Rénia et al., 2018). The burden of multiple infections can further compromise health, increase morbidity, and reduce overall quality of life.

Addressing the long-term effects of repeated malaria infections requires a comprehensive approach to malaria control and prevention. This includes strategies such as vector control, access to prompt and effective treatment, preventive measures like insecticide-treated bed nets and intermittent preventive treatment in pregnancy, and efforts to reduce malaria transmission rates.

Investing in long-term solutions, strengthening healthcare systems, and promoting socio-economic development in malaria-endemic regions are essential for mitigating the health and well-being consequences of repeated malaria infections.

Chapter 5. Economic Impact of Malaria in West Africa

5.1 Productivity losses due to malaria-related illnesses and deaths

Malaria-related illnesses and deaths have a significant impact on productivity, leading to economic losses in malaria-endemic regions like West Africa. The following discussion highlights the productivity losses associated with malaria, supported by relevant in-text citations:

5.1.1 Lost workdays and reduced productivity:

Malaria-related illnesses indeed lead to lost workdays and reduced productivity, as highlighted by Gallup and Sachs (2001).

The debilitating symptoms of malaria, including high fever, fatigue, and body aches, can render individuals unable to carry out their regular work activities. This results in missed workdays, where individuals are unable to attend their jobs due to the severity of their illness. These missed workdays not only impact the affected individuals but also result in economic losses for employers and the wider economy.

Even when individuals with malaria are able to continue working, the symptoms can significantly reduce their ability to perform at full capacity. Fatigue and weakness can limit physical exertion, impairing individuals' ability to engage in physically demanding tasks. Cognitive symptoms, such as difficulty concentrating and impaired memory, can hinder individuals' ability to complete complex or mentally demanding work.

The reduced capacity to work and the impact on productivity have broader implications for individuals, families, and communities. Decreased productivity due to malaria-related illnesses can result in reduced income for affected individuals, limiting their ability to meet their basic needs and potentially pushing them further into poverty. At the community level, the cumulative effect of reduced productivity can hinder economic growth and development.

Addressing the impact of malaria on lost workdays and productivity requires effective prevention and control strategies. Access to prompt and affordable diagnosis and treatment of malaria cases is crucial to minimize the duration and severity of illness, allowing individuals to return to work more quickly. Prevention measures, such as the use of insecticide-treated bed nets and indoor residual spraying, can help reduce the incidence of malaria and its associated impact on productivity.

Furthermore, raising awareness about malaria symptoms and prevention measures can help individuals take appropriate actions to protect themselves and seek early treatment when necessary. Supportive workplace policies, such as sick leave provisions and flexible working arrangements, can also contribute to reducing the impact of malaria on lost workdays and productivity.

Frequent episodes of malaria can create a cycle of recurring illness, recovery, and reduced work productivity, affecting both individuals and their communities.

5.1.2 Economic impact on households and communities:

Malaria-related illnesses impose a significant financial burden on affected individuals and their families, as highlighted by Littrell et al. (2013). The costs associated with malaria treatment, including expenses for healthcare services, diagnostic tests, and medications, can strain household resources. Additionally, transportation costs to access healthcare facilities and the need for caretakers or additional support during illness further contribute to the economic hardships faced by affected households.

Furthermore, the loss of income due to missed workdays resulting from malaria-related illnesses adds to the economic burden. When individuals are unable to work due to the severity of their illness or reduced productivity, it directly impacts their earning potential and limits their ability to meet their financial obligations and provide for their families.

The economic impact of malaria extends beyond the individual household level and can have broader implications for communities and local economies. Reduced productivity and economic losses at the household level can have ripple effects on the overall community. As more households face economic hardships due to malaria-related illnesses, the local economy may suffer as well, particularly in settings where malaria is endemic and a significant proportion of the population is affected.

The economic burden of malaria not only affects the affected households and communities but also poses challenges to economic development and poverty reduction efforts. The cumulative effect of reduced productivity, increased healthcare expenditures, and the perpetuation of a cycle of poverty can hinder overall socio-economic progress in malaria-endemic regions.

Addressing the economic impact of malaria on households and communities requires comprehensive interventions. This includes improving access to affordable and quality healthcare services, implementing preventive measures such as the use of insecticide-treated bed nets and indoor residual spraying, and promoting early diagnosis and prompt treatment of malaria cases. Additionally, supportive policies at the national and community levels that address income loss, provide financial protection, and support economic resilience can help alleviate the economic burden faced by affected households and communities.

Table 4: Approximate cost ranges for various components related to malaria treatment and healthcare

Cost Category	Approximate Cost Range (in USD)	Data Source(s)
Consultation Fee	$5 - $20	Various local health facilities and surveys
Diagnostic Tests	$2 - $10	Studies on healthcare costs in West Africa
Antimalarial Drugs	$1 - $10 per course of treatment	National health reports and studies on medication costs
Hospitalization (if required)	$50 - $200 per day	Research on hospitalization costs and fees
Transportation Costs	$5 - $50 (varies with distance)	Studies on healthcare access and transportation expenses

The table provides an overview of the approximate cost ranges for various components related to malaria treatment and healthcare in West Africa. The cost categories include consultation fees, diagnostic tests, antimalarial drugs, hospitalization (if required), and transportation costs.

• • • •

THE IMPACT OF MALARIA ON THE SOCIAL-ECONOMIC DEVELOPMENT OF WEST AFRICA

HERE IS A SUMMARY LIST of studies that have explored the costs associated with malaria treatment, including expenses for healthcare services, diagnostic tests, and medications:

Table 5: List of studies that have explored the costs associated with malaria

Study	Country	Data Collection Period	Key Findings
Chizema-Kawesha et al., 2017	Zambia	2012-2014	Out-of-pocket costs for malaria treatment were a significant financial burden for households.
Galactionova et al., 2014	Mozambique	2010-2011	Malaria treatment costs accounted for a substantial portion of healthcare expenditures in households.
Onwujekwe et al., 2010	Nigeria	2008-2009	Households in rural areas faced higher direct and indirect costs for malaria treatment compared to urban areas.
Wiseman et al., 2019	Ghana	2015-2017	The economic burden of malaria treatment was significant, with households experiencing financial hardship.
O'Connell et al., 2019	Burkina Faso	2015-2016	Malaria treatment costs were high, and affordability was a significant challenge for households.
Tine et al., 2014	Senegal	2009-2010	Direct and indirect costs of malaria treatment accounted for a considerable proportion of household income.
Toda et al., 2020	Sierra Leone	2017-2018	Malaria treatment costs were associated with catastrophic health expenditure for many households.

Please note that this is not an exhaustive list, and there are numerous other studies available on the topic. The studies mentioned above highlight the financial burden of malaria treatment and provide insights into the costs incurred by households in various countries in sub-Saharan Africa.

It is essential to refer to each specific study for more comprehensive information on the methodology, sample size, cost components assessed, and the context in which the research was conducted.

5.1.3 Impact on agricultural productivity:

Malaria-related illnesses can indeed have a detrimental impact on agricultural productivity, as emphasized by Sachs and Malaney (2002). Here are some impacts to consider:

5.1.3.1 Effect on Farmers' Work Capacity and Agricultural Output

IN MALARIA-ENDEMIC regions where agriculture is a primary livelihood, farmers affected by malaria may experience reduced work capacity due to the debilitating symptoms of the disease. High fevers, fatigue, and body aches can limit individuals' physical endurance and ability to engage in strenuous agricultural activities. As a result, farmers may have difficulty working for extended periods, leading to decreased agricultural output and lower incomes.

5.1.3.2 Reduced Work Capacity among Farmers in Endemic Regions

THE REDUCED WORK CAPACITY of affected farmers can have broader implications for food security and economic well-being. Decreased agricultural productivity not only affects the individual farmers but also has an impact on the overall agricultural sector and local economies. Malaria-related illnesses among farmers can lead to lower yields, reduced crop quality, and disrupted farming schedules, affecting the availability and affordability of food in malaria-endemic areas.

5.1.3.3 Implications for Economic Growth, Poverty, and Food Insecurity in Endemic Regions

THE ECONOMIC GROWTH of malaria-endemic regions heavily relies on the agricultural sector. Decreased productivity in agriculture due to malaria-related illnesses can hinder economic development and perpetuate a cycle of poverty in these areas. The income loss experienced by farmers and the resulting economic impact on communities further contribute to food insecurity and limited access to basic necessities.

Addressing the impact of malaria on agricultural productivity requires comprehensive approaches. Preventive measures such as the use of insecticide-treated bed nets and indoor residual spraying can help reduce malaria transmission among farmers. Timely diagnosis and treatment of malaria cases, along with supportive healthcare services, can minimize the duration and severity of illness, allowing farmers to maintain their work capacity.

Furthermore, providing access to agricultural resources, including improved farming techniques, tools, and irrigation systems, can help enhance productivity and resilience among farmers in malaria-endemic areas. Promoting agricultural diversification and value-added activities can also contribute to economic growth and reduce the vulnerability of communities to malaria-related disruptions.

5.1.4 Implications for economic development:

The productivity losses resulting from malaria-related illnesses and deaths pose significant obstacles to economic development in regions affected by the disease. Studies by Gallup and Sachs (2001) have shown the detrimental effects of malaria on productivity, while Sachs and Malaney (2002) highlight the broader economic implications, including reduced investments, limited opportunities for economic growth, and challenges in poverty reduction. Addressing malaria transmission and reducing productivity losses are crucial for achieving sustainable socio-economic development in these regions.

5.1.4.1 Comprehensive Approach to Malaria Control:

EFFORTS TO CONTROL malaria and minimize productivity losses require a comprehensive approach. This includes implementing a range of interventions such as the distribution and promotion of insecticide-treated bed nets to protect individuals from mosquito bites, indoor residual spraying to reduce mosquito populations, prompt diagnosis and effective treatment of malaria cases, and ongoing research and development for new interventions and strategies. These measures are essential for breaking the cycle of malaria transmission and mitigating its impact on productivity.

5.1.4.2 Role of Malaria Control in Economic Development:

INVESTING IN MALARIA control programs yields multiple benefits beyond improving individual health and well-being. By reducing productivity losses associated with malaria-related illnesses, these programs contribute to economic development in affected regions. When individuals are healthy and able to work, agricultural and other economic activities can thrive, attracting investments and fostering economic growth. Moreover, the reduction of malaria cases and related healthcare costs can free up resources for other development initiatives, such as education and infrastructure improvements, further fueling socio-economic progress.

5.1.4.3 Promoting Sustainable Growth:

ACHIEVING SUSTAINABLE socio-economic development requires a long-term perspective on malaria control. By implementing effective prevention and treatment strategies, communities can break free from the cycle of malaria transmission and its associated productivity losses. Sustainable economic growth depends on maintaining low malaria transmission rates, ensuring access to quality healthcare services, and investing in research and development to continuously improve malaria control measures.

5.2 Impact on agriculture and food security

Malaria has a significant impact on agriculture and food security in malaria-endemic regions like West Africa. The following discussion highlights the effects of malaria on agricultural productivity and food security, supported by relevant in-text citations:

5.2.1 Decreased agricultural productivity:

Malaria-related illnesses can indeed lead to reduced work capacity and productivity among agricultural workers, as highlighted by Sachs and Malaney (2002). The symptoms associated with malaria can severely impact farmers' ability to carry out their farming activities. Farmers affected by malaria may experience symptoms such as fatigue, weakness, and other flu-like symptoms that can significantly limit their ability to engage in various farming tasks, including land preparation, planting, and harvesting (Littrell et al., 2013).

The debilitating symptoms of malaria, including fatigue and weakness, can result in decreased productivity and efficiency among agricultural workers. Sachs and Malaney (2002) emphasize that the reduced work capacity resulting from malaria contributes to decreased agricultural output. This decrease in productivity directly affects the incomes of farmers, as lower yields and disrupted farming schedules can lead to financial losses. The economic losses experienced by individual farmers extend to their communities, as the agricultural sector plays a vital role in local economies.

The reduced agricultural productivity resulting from malaria has significant implications for both farmers and their communities. Lower agricultural output leads to lower incomes and economic losses. This not only affects the livelihoods of individual farmers but also impacts the overall economic well-being of their communities. In malaria-endemic areas where agriculture is a primary livelihood, decreased agricultural productivity can lead to limited access to food, higher food prices, and overall economic stagnation (Sachs & Malaney, 2002).

Addressing the impact of malaria on agricultural productivity requires comprehensive interventions. Preventive measures such as the use of insecticide-treated bed nets and indoor residual spraying can reduce malaria transmission and protect agricultural workers from mosquito bites. Access to prompt and affordable diagnosis and treatment of malaria cases is crucial in minimizing the duration and severity of illness among farmers, allowing them to maintain their work capacity and productivity (Littrell et al., 2013).

Investing in agricultural infrastructure, resources, and improved farming techniques can also enhance productivity and resilience among farmers in malaria-endemic regions. Providing training and education on malaria prevention and control, as well as promoting sustainable agricultural practices, can further contribute to mitigating the impact of malaria on agricultural productivity.

5.2.2 Impact on labor availability:

Malaria can indeed have a significant impact on labor availability in the agricultural sectors, as highlighted by Sachs and Malaney (2002). The prevalence of malaria-related illnesses among agricultural workers can result in absenteeism and reduced work capacity, leading to labor shortages.

Malaria-related absenteeism and decreased work capacity can have detrimental effects on the agricultural workforce, particularly during peak agricultural seasons. Littrell et al. (2013) note that the symptoms associated with malaria, such as fatigue, weakness, and other flu-like symptoms, can limit the ability of affected individuals to carry out their farming activities. This can result in labor shortages, as agricultural workers are unable to participate fully or consistently in farming activities, including land preparation, planting, and harvesting.

The labor shortages caused by malaria-related absenteeism and reduced work capacity can disrupt the timely completion of farming activities. This can have consequences for agricultural production, leading to delays in planting or harvesting, lower yields, and overall reduced productivity in the agricultural sector. The lack of labor availability during crucial periods can affect the quality of agricultural output and limit the capacity of farmers to meet market demands.

The impact of malaria on labor availability in the agricultural sector has broader implications for food security, income generation, and economic development. Labor shortages can lead to decreased agricultural output, affecting food availability and affordability in malaria-endemic areas. Additionally, lower agricultural productivity can result in reduced incomes for farmers and their communities, perpetuating the cycle of poverty.

Addressing the impact of malaria on labor availability requires comprehensive approaches. Preventive measures, such as the use of insecticide-treated bed nets and indoor residual spraying, can reduce malaria transmission and protect agricultural workers from mosquito bites. Timely diagnosis and treatment of malaria cases, along with supportive healthcare services, can minimize the duration and severity of illness among agricultural workers, allowing them to maintain their work capacity.

Furthermore, investments in improving healthcare infrastructure, access to healthcare services, and the availability of effective antimalarial treatments are crucial in reducing the burden of malaria-related illnesses and preventing labor shortages in the agricultural sector. Promoting awareness and education on malaria prevention and control measures among agricultural workers can also contribute to minimizing the impact of malaria on labor availability.

5.2.3 Food security:

Malaria can indeed undermine food security, as it has various impacts on agricultural productivity and access to food. Littrell et al. (2013) highlight that malaria-related illnesses can reduce agricultural productivity, which in turn can limit the availability of food supplies. Decreased agricultural output due to malaria can result in insufficient food supplies for local consumption and trade, exacerbating food shortages and raising prices (Sachs & Malaney, 2002).

The reduced agricultural productivity resulting from malaria-related absenteeism and decreased work capacity can lead to decreased food production. This can have severe implications for local communities and contribute to food shortages. Insufficient food supplies can directly affect food security by limiting access to an adequate and diverse diet, particularly for vulnerable populations.

Furthermore, malaria-related illnesses can impact household incomes, limiting the purchasing power of individuals to acquire food. The economic burden of malaria, including healthcare expenses and lost income due to missed workdays, can further exacerbate the vulnerability to food insecurity among affected households. Limited financial resources can restrict individuals' ability to purchase sufficient and nutritious food, increasing the risk of malnutrition.

Addressing the impact of malaria on food security requires a multifaceted approach. Preventive measures, such as the use of insecticide-treated bed nets and indoor residual spraying, can reduce malaria transmission and protect agricultural workers from mosquito bites, contributing to sustained agricultural productivity. Timely diagnosis and treatment of malaria cases, along with supportive healthcare services, can minimize the duration and severity of illness among individuals, reducing the economic burden and enhancing their ability to maintain their livelihoods.

Additionally, promoting sustainable agricultural practices, improving access to agricultural resources and technologies, and investing in irrigation systems and storage facilities can enhance agricultural productivity and resilience, ensuring a more stable food supply. Enhancing farmers' capacity through training and education on improved farming techniques and diversification can also contribute to increased food production and security.

5.2.4 Interactions with other factors:

Malaria interacts with other agricultural challenges, such as climate change and water management issues, leading to compounding effects on food security. (Littrell et al., 2013).

Environmental factors that favor malaria transmission, such as stagnant water, can coincide with conditions necessary for agricultural productivity, creating complex challenges for farmers in malaria-endemic areas.

Addressing malaria's impact on agriculture and food security requires integrated approaches. This includes implementing malaria control interventions, promoting agricultural practices resilient to malaria risks, improving access to healthcare for farmers, and enhancing agricultural extension services to raise awareness about malaria prevention measures.

By addressing the nexus between malaria, agriculture, and food security, sustainable solutions can be developed to mitigate the adverse effects of malaria on agricultural productivity and promote food availability and stability in malaria-endemic regions.

5.3 Analysis of healthcare costs and expenditures related to malaria treatment and prevention

Healthcare costs and expenditures related to malaria treatment and prevention pose a significant economic burden on individuals, households, healthcare systems, and governments in West Africa. The following analysis explores the financial implications of malaria in terms of treatment costs and prevention strategies, supported by relevant information and studies:

5.3.1 Treatment costs:

Malaria treatment costs encompass various components, including expenses associated with diagnosis, antimalarial drugs, hospitalization, and follow-up care, as emphasized by Chuma et al. (2006). Individuals affected by malaria in malaria-endemic regions often seek healthcare services to receive the necessary treatment, leading to direct out-of-pocket payments. These out-of-pocket payments for malaria treatment can be particularly burdensome for low-income households, resulting in financial hardships.

The costs of malaria treatment can impose a significant financial burden on affected individuals and their families, potentially pushing them into poverty. Chuma et al. (2006) highlight that low-income households may struggle to afford the expenses associated with malaria diagnosis, medication, and hospitalization. These financial hardships can further exacerbate the cycle of poverty, limiting the resources available for other essential needs, such as food, education, and basic amenities.

The economic burden of malaria treatment extends beyond individual households. The cumulative costs of treating malaria cases within a community or region can have broader implications for the healthcare system and the overall economy. The financial strain placed on healthcare facilities and resources to manage malaria cases can divert resources from other essential healthcare services.

Addressing the cost burden of malaria treatment requires comprehensive approaches. Efforts should focus on improving access to affordable and effective antimalarial drugs, ensuring availability and accessibility of diagnostic tools, and promoting cost-effective treatment options. Strengthening health systems and social protection mechanisms can help alleviate the financial burden on affected individuals and households, particularly those from low-income backgrounds.

Additionally, investments in preventive measures, such as the use of insecticide-treated bed nets and indoor residual spraying, can contribute to reducing the incidence of malaria cases and the subsequent need for treatment. By preventing malaria infections, these interventions can help alleviate the financial strain on individuals, households, and healthcare systems.

5.3.2 Health system costs:

Malaria indeed places a strain on healthcare systems, as highlighted by Chima et al. (2010). The burden of malaria increases the demand for healthcare services, including diagnosis, treatment, and follow-up care. Healthcare facilities and providers need to allocate resources to meet this increased demand and effectively manage malaria cases.

Health systems must allocate resources for the training of healthcare providers to ensure they have the knowledge and skills necessary to diagnose and treat malaria cases. This includes training on proper case management, use of diagnostic tools, and administration of antimalarial drugs. Adequate training enables healthcare providers to deliver quality care and improve treatment outcomes for malaria patients.

In addition to healthcare provider training, health systems must allocate resources for the procurement of antimalarial drugs and other treatment supplies. Ensuring a steady supply of effective antimalarial medications is crucial for the prompt treatment of malaria cases and reducing the burden of the disease. Diagnostic facilities, such as microscopy or rapid diagnostic tests, also require resources for maintenance and regular supply to enable accurate and timely diagnosis of malaria infections.

The strain on healthcare systems posed by malaria underscores the importance of resource allocation and effective management. Health systems need to prioritize the allocation of resources to malaria control and management, taking into account the high prevalence and impact of the disease. This includes strengthening infrastructure, supply chains, and surveillance systems to effectively respond to malaria cases and provide timely and appropriate care.

Furthermore, investments in health system strengthening, such as improving healthcare infrastructure, expanding access to essential medicines, and strengthening surveillance and reporting systems, are essential in effectively managing malaria cases and reducing the burden on healthcare systems.

The costs associated with expanding and strengthening healthcare infrastructure to address malaria burden add to the overall healthcare expenditures.

5.3.3 Prevention strategies and costs:

Malaria prevention strategies, such as the distribution of insecticide-treated bed nets (ITNs), indoor residual spraying (IRS), and intermittent preventive treatment in pregnancy (IPTp), play a crucial role in reducing the burden of malaria. However, these prevention interventions also come with associated costs, as emphasized by Owusu-Addo et al. (2018).

The procurement, distribution, and maintenance of ITNs and IRS require financial resources and logistical efforts from healthcare systems and governments. The costs involved in manufacturing or purchasing ITNs, distributing them to communities, and ensuring their regular maintenance and replacement add to the overall expenses of malaria prevention efforts. Similarly, indoor residual spraying programs require the procurement of insecticides, training of personnel, and ongoing efforts to implement and sustain spraying activities. Furthermore, the provision of intermittent preventive treatment in pregnancy (IPTp), which involves administering antimalarial drugs to pregnant women, also incurs costs related to drug procurement and healthcare delivery.

It is essential to consider the costs associated with malaria prevention interventions alongside treatment costs when assessing the overall economic burden of malaria. While prevention strategies require upfront investments, they are cost-effective in the long run by reducing the incidence of malaria cases, hospitalizations, and treatment expenses. Additionally, these prevention interventions contribute to improved health outcomes, reduced productivity losses, and enhanced quality of life for individuals and communities affected by malaria.

To ensure the sustainability of malaria prevention strategies, it is crucial to prioritize resource allocation and develop robust financing mechanisms. Governments, in collaboration with international partners and organizations, need to invest in the procurement, distribution, and maintenance of prevention interventions. This includes strategic planning, budget allocation, and monitoring and evaluation to ensure the effective implementation of prevention programs. Furthermore, efforts should be made to increase access to prevention interventions, particularly among vulnerable populations, to maximize their impact in reducing malaria transmission.

5.3.4 Socioeconomic impact:

High healthcare costs and expenditures related to malaria can lead to catastrophic health spending, where households are forced to spend a significant portion of their income on healthcare, compromising their overall well-being. (Owusu-Addo et al., 2018).

The economic burden of malaria can limit households' ability to invest in education, nutrition, and other essential needs, perpetuating a cycle of poverty and hindering socio-economic development. (Chuma et al., 2006).

Efforts to address the healthcare costs and expenditures related to malaria involve a multi-pronged approach. This includes reducing treatment costs through affordable access to quality healthcare services, improving healthcare financing mechanisms, and strengthening health systems to provide comprehensive and cost-effective malaria prevention and treatment services.

Furthermore, investing in cost-effective prevention strategies, such as expanding the coverage of ITNs, implementing IRS programs, and promoting IPTp, can help reduce the overall burden of malaria and alleviate the economic impact on individuals and healthcare systems.

5.4 Examination of the indirect costs of malaria

Malaria imposes significant indirect costs on affected regions, including detrimental effects on educational attainment and the tourism industry. The following analysis explores the indirect costs of malaria and their impact, supported by relevant information and studies:

5.4.1 Reduced educational attainment:

Malaria-related illnesses can have a significant impact on educational attainment, as highlighted by Brooker et al. (2000). The debilitating symptoms of malaria, such as fever, fatigue, and weakness, can lead to absenteeism from school, affecting children's regular attendance and educational continuity. Frequent or prolonged absences due to malaria episodes can disrupt the learning process and hinder academic performance.

Moreover, the cognitive impairments resulting from malaria infections can further hinder children's learning abilities and intellectual development, leading to lower educational attainment. Fernando et al. (2016) emphasize the long-term effects of malaria on cognitive function, including memory deficits, attention problems, and impaired information processing. These cognitive impairments can have a cumulative effect, impacting children's ability to comprehend new concepts, engage in complex reasoning, and achieve academic milestones.

The reduced educational attainment resulting from malaria infections contributes to the perpetuation of the cycle of poverty. Limited access to quality education and lower educational achievements limit individuals' opportunities for socio-economic advancement. Without sufficient education, individuals may face barriers in accessing higher-paying jobs, acquiring new skills, and breaking free from the constraints of poverty. This, in turn, can hinder overall human capital development and impede socio-economic progress at both the individual and societal levels.

Efforts to mitigate the impact of malaria on educational attainment require a multi-faceted approach. Strengthening malaria prevention and control measures, such as widespread distribution of insecticide-treated bed nets in malaria-endemic areas, can reduce the incidence of malaria infections and minimize school disruptions due to illness. Additionally, improving access to prompt and effective treatment for malaria cases can help minimize the duration and severity of episodes, reducing absenteeism and promoting regular school attendance.

Furthermore, targeted interventions are needed to support affected students and mitigate the cognitive impacts of malaria on learning. This may include implementing catch-up programs, providing additional educational support and resources, and raising awareness among educators, parents, and communities about the importance of early detection and treatment of malaria.

5.4.2 Impact on workforce productivity:

Malaria-related illnesses have a significant impact on workforce productivity, as highlighted by Gallup and Sachs (2001). The debilitating symptoms of malaria, such as fever, fatigue, and body aches, can lead to decreased work capacity and absenteeism from work. Individuals affected by malaria may be unable to perform their job duties at full capacity or may need to take time off work to recover from the illness. These factors contribute to reduced workforce productivity.

The impact of malaria on workforce productivity extends beyond individual workers to various sectors of the economy. In malaria-endemic regions, where a significant portion of the population is at risk of the disease, the collective effect of decreased productivity can be substantial. Industries such as agriculture, construction, and manufacturing, which heavily rely on manual labor, may experience significant disruptions due to malaria-related absenteeism and reduced work capacity.

The negative impact on workforce productivity has broader implications for economic growth and development. Limited human resources due to malaria-related illnesses can hinder the ability of businesses and industries to meet production targets and fulfill market demands. This, in turn, can lead to decreased profitability, reduced competitiveness, and missed economic opportunities. The cumulative effect of reduced workforce productivity across various sectors can hamper overall economic growth and impede progress in malaria-endemic regions.

Addressing the impact of malaria on workforce productivity requires comprehensive strategies that encompass both prevention and treatment. Preventive measures such as the distribution of insecticide-treated bed nets, indoor residual spraying, and targeted interventions for high-risk populations can reduce the incidence of malaria and minimize the impact on workforce productivity. Prompt diagnosis and effective treatment of malaria cases are also crucial to ensure swift recovery and minimize workdays lost due to illness.

In addition to prevention and treatment, raising awareness about malaria prevention and encouraging early treatment-seeking behaviors among individuals and communities are important. Education campaigns and workplace interventions can promote knowledge about malaria prevention measures, encourage the use of preventive measures, and support prompt treatment-seeking behaviors when symptoms arise. Employers can also play a role by providing supportive workplace environments, such as access to healthcare services and flexible sick leave policies, to accommodate employees affected by malaria.

Malaria, as a vector-borne disease, can have a significant impact on the tourism industry in endemic regions. Concerns about the transmission of malaria can deter tourists from visiting affected areas, resulting in reduced revenue and job opportunities in the tourism sector. This is emphasized by Ettling et al. (1992), who highlight the association between malaria-endemicity and decreased tourism.

The perception of malaria risk plays a crucial role in tourists' decision-making process. Travelers may choose to avoid or postpone trips to malaria-endemic regions due to concerns about contracting the disease. The potential health risks associated with malaria, such as the need for preventive measures and the possibility of experiencing malaria-related complications, can create a sense of uncertainty and anxiety among tourists. This, in turn, can lead to decreased tourist arrivals and economic losses for the tourism industry.

Efforts to control and prevent malaria are essential to reassure tourists and promote sustainable tourism in malaria-endemic regions. Vector control measures, such as the use of insecticide-treated bed nets and indoor residual spraying, can reduce the mosquito population and lower the risk of malaria transmission. Effective treatment and prompt diagnosis of malaria cases are also critical in minimizing the likelihood of tourists contracting the disease during their visit.

Collaboration between the tourism industry, local communities, and public health authorities is crucial in implementing comprehensive malaria control and prevention strategies. Public awareness campaigns, targeted at both tourists and local populations, can educate individuals about the measures taken to reduce the risk of malaria transmission. These efforts can help alleviate tourists' concerns, promote a positive perception of the destination, and encourage travel to malaria-endemic areas.

Furthermore, investing in healthcare infrastructure and ensuring access to quality healthcare services in tourism hotspots can enhance the safety and well-being of tourists. The availability of effective diagnosis and treatment facilities can provide reassurance to travelers and contribute to the overall health security of the destination.

5.4.4 Economic impact:

The indirect costs of malaria, including reduced educational attainment and tourism decline, have long-term economic consequences for affected regions. (Ettling et al., 1992).

Lower educational attainment limits the pool of skilled labor, while reduced tourism reduces revenue and employment opportunities.

These economic impacts can hinder socio-economic development, perpetuate poverty, and widen the development gap between malaria-endemic regions and non-endemic regions.

Addressing the indirect costs of malaria requires comprehensive strategies that go beyond healthcare interventions. Investing in quality education, implementing malaria control measures to reduce school absenteeism, and promoting public awareness about the disease's prevention and treatment are vital for mitigating the indirect costs of malaria on educational attainment.

Furthermore, strengthening malaria control efforts, improving healthcare infrastructure, and enhancing the perception of safety in malaria-endemic regions can help restore and attract tourism, boosting economic growth and development.

By recognizing and addressing the indirect costs of malaria, governments, policymakers, and international organizations can implement holistic approaches to malaria control and prevention, leading to improved educational outcomes, enhanced workforce productivity, and sustainable economic development.

Chapter 6. Social Impact of Malaria in West Africa

6.1 Social consequences of malaria

Malaria not only has health and economic implications but also leads to social consequences, including stigma and discrimination. The following discussion explores the social impact of malaria:

6.1.1 Stigma associated with malaria:

Malaria stigma is a significant social consequence associated with the disease, as highlighted by Tanner et al. (2015). Malaria is often stigmatized due to its association with poverty, unsanitary conditions, and misconceptions about its transmission. The perception that malaria is a result of personal negligence or unclean living conditions can lead to blame and social exclusion of individuals and communities affected by the disease.

Stigma surrounding malaria can have detrimental effects on the well-being and social fabric of affected individuals and communities. People affected by malaria may face discrimination, rejection, and social isolation, leading to feelings of shame, guilt, and low self-esteem. This can contribute to psychological distress and mental health problems, further exacerbating the burden of the disease on affected individuals.

Stigma can also impede access to healthcare services for individuals and families affected by malaria. Fear of discrimination or negative judgment may deter individuals from seeking timely diagnosis and treatment, leading to delayed or inadequate care. Molyneux et al. (2018) highlight the negative impact of stigma on healthcare-seeking behavior for malaria, which can result in increased morbidity and mortality.

Addressing malaria stigma requires comprehensive strategies that focus on education, awareness, and community engagement. Public health campaigns can play a crucial role in dispelling misconceptions about malaria transmission, emphasizing the shared responsibility in preventing and controlling the disease, and promoting empathy and support for affected individuals. These campaigns should aim to reduce the blame and discrimination associated with malaria and foster a supportive environment for affected individuals and communities. Community engagement and involvement of local leaders and influencers are also important in challenging and changing social norms and attitudes towards malaria. By promoting understanding, empathy, and acceptance, communities can create an inclusive and supportive environment for those affected by malaria.

Furthermore, efforts to improve access to healthcare services, including diagnosis, treatment, and prevention, can help address the barriers caused by stigma. Making healthcare services accessible, affordable, and non-discriminatory can encourage individuals to seek timely care without fear of social repercussions.

6.1.2 Discrimination and socioeconomic disparities:

The burden of malaria is often concentrated in marginalized communities that face multiple socioeconomic challenges, including limited access to healthcare, clean water, and sanitation facilities. This is highlighted by Tanner et al. (2015), who emphasize that malaria burden tends to be higher in communities with lower socioeconomic status.

Discrimination and stigmatization related to malaria can exacerbate existing socioeconomic disparities, further perpetuating inequalities. Individuals and communities affected by malaria may face discrimination in various aspects of life, including education and employment opportunities. Stigma can hinder educational attainment, limiting individuals' chances for socioeconomic advancement. Additionally, discrimination in the workplace can result in reduced employment opportunities and income disparities.

The social consequences of malaria, including stigma and discrimination, can contribute to a cycle of poverty and vulnerability in affected regions. The combination of health and socioeconomic challenges makes it difficult for individuals and communities to break free from the cycle of poverty and improve their overall well-being. This perpetuates inequalities and hinders socioeconomic development in malaria-endemic areas.

Addressing discrimination and socioeconomic disparities related to malaria requires a comprehensive approach that focuses on improving access to healthcare, education, and economic opportunities. Efforts should be made to ensure equitable access to healthcare services, including malaria prevention, diagnosis, and treatment. Investing in infrastructure development, such as clean water and sanitation facilities, can also contribute to reducing malaria burden and socioeconomic disparities.

Furthermore, addressing the root causes of discrimination and stigma associated with malaria requires community engagement, awareness campaigns, and advocacy for social inclusion. By promoting understanding, empathy, and equal opportunities, communities can work towards breaking the cycle of poverty and vulnerability and fostering a more equitable and inclusive society.

6.1.3 Impact on mental health and well-being:

The social stigma associated with malaria can have a profound impact on the mental health and well-being of individuals and communities affected by the disease. Molyneux et al. (2018) highlight that the stigma surrounding malaria can result in feelings of shame, embarrassment, and social isolation. Individuals may experience internalized stigma, perceiving themselves as flawed or unworthy due to their association with the disease. This can lead to psychological distress, including anxiety and depression, and have long-lasting effects on mental well-being.

The fear of being stigmatized can also discourage individuals from seeking timely diagnosis and treatment for malaria. Tanner et al. (2015) emphasize that the fear of social repercussions, such as being blamed or ostracized, may create barriers to healthcare-seeking behavior. This can lead to delayed or inadequate care, resulting in worsened health outcomes for individuals and increased transmission risk within the community.

The impact of malaria-related stigma on mental health and well-being highlights the need for comprehensive approaches in malaria control and prevention efforts. It is essential to address the social and psychological dimensions of the disease to mitigate the negative consequences on mental health. This includes raising awareness about malaria, combating misconceptions and stereotypes, and promoting empathy and support for affected individuals and communities.

Creating safe spaces for open dialogue and reducing the fear of stigma can encourage individuals to seek timely diagnosis and treatment. Accessible and confidential healthcare services that prioritize non-discriminatory and patient-centered care are crucial in ensuring that individuals feel comfortable and supported in seeking necessary care for malaria.

Furthermore, integrating mental health support into malaria control programs is important. This can involve training healthcare providers to recognize and address the psychological impact of malaria on individuals and offering psychosocial support to those affected by the disease.

6.1.4 Gender-related implications:

Malaria can have gender-specific implications, particularly for women, due to existing societal norms and gender inequalities. Tanner et al. (2015) note that women often bear a disproportionate burden of caregiving responsibilities for family members affected by malaria. This can include taking care of sick family members, seeking medical treatment, and managing household tasks, which can result in increased physical and emotional strain on women.

Gender inequalities can further compound the impact of malaria on women. Societal norms and expectations may limit women's access to resources, healthcare services, and opportunities for education and economic empowerment. Women may face barriers in accessing timely and appropriate malaria prevention, diagnosis, and treatment due to factors such as limited decision-making power, lack of control over financial resources, and limited mobility.

The gender-specific implications of malaria highlight the need for gender-responsive approaches in malaria control and prevention efforts. It is crucial to address gender inequalities and empower women to actively participate in decision-making processes related to their health and the health of their families. This can involve providing targeted support, such as ensuring access to healthcare services, promoting education and awareness about malaria, and creating economic opportunities for women.

Integrating gender perspectives into malaria programs can help identify and address the unique challenges faced by women, ensuring that their needs are adequately met. This can involve engaging women in the design and implementation of malaria control strategies, fostering gender equality and women's empowerment, and addressing structural barriers that limit women's access to resources and opportunities.

Addressing the social consequences of malaria requires comprehensive strategies that focus not only on healthcare interventions but also on promoting social inclusion and combating stigma. This includes raising awareness about the causes and transmission of malaria, dispelling misconceptions, and promoting community engagement and support for affected individuals and families.

Moreover, efforts to improve access to education, healthcare, and economic opportunities can contribute to reducing the social disparities and discrimination associated with malaria. Integrating malaria control programs with broader social development initiatives is crucial for addressing the social consequences and achieving sustainable progress in malaria-endemic regions.

6.2 Examination of the gender dimensions of malaria

Malaria affects women and girls in unique ways due to biological, socio-cultural, and economic factors. Understanding the gender dimensions of malaria is crucial for developing targeted interventions and addressing the specific challenges faced by women and girls. The following examination highlights the effects of malaria on women and girls, supported by relevant in-text citations:

6.2.1 Maternal health and pregnancy:

Pregnant women in malaria-endemic regions face specific challenges and risks associated with malaria infection. Dellicour et al. (2017) highlight that pregnant women are at an increased risk of malaria infection and related complications compared to the general population. Malaria during pregnancy can lead to severe anemia, low birth weight, preterm delivery, and maternal mortality. These adverse outcomes pose significant risks to the health and well-being of both the mother and the developing fetus.

Malaria in pregnancy can have long-term health consequences for both the mother and the child. Desai et al. (2018) emphasize that malaria infections during pregnancy can contribute to impaired fetal growth, developmental delays, and increased risk of chronic diseases later in life. These effects highlight the importance of addressing malaria in pregnancy as a critical component of maternal and child health.

However, women in malaria-endemic regions often face challenges in accessing adequate antenatal care services and interventions. Dellicour et al. (2017) note that limited access to healthcare facilities, including antenatal care clinics, can hinder early detection and prompt treatment of malaria in pregnant women. This, in turn, exacerbates the risks associated with malaria in pregnancy and increases the likelihood of adverse outcomes.

To mitigate the risks associated with malaria in pregnancy, comprehensive approaches are needed. These include integrating malaria prevention and treatment measures into routine antenatal care services, ensuring access to insecticide-treated bed nets and preventive medications, and providing regular monitoring and follow-up for pregnant women. Strengthening healthcare systems and improving access to quality antenatal care services in malaria-endemic regions are crucial in reducing the burden of malaria on maternal and child health.

6.2.2 Caregiving responsibilities:

Women and girls in malaria-endemic regions often bear a significant burden of caregiving responsibilities for family members affected by malaria. Kilian et al. (2016) highlight that women assume caregiving roles, including providing care for children and other family members who are sick with malaria. This responsibility can have implications for women's time allocation, educational opportunities, and economic participation.

The caregiving responsibilities associated with malaria can affect women's ability to engage in income-generating activities and pursue educational opportunities. Littrell et al. (2013) emphasize that caring for malaria-affected individuals, particularly children, can limit women's availability and capacity to participate in the workforce or seek educational advancement. This perpetuates gender inequalities and restricts women's opportunities for economic empowerment and personal development.

The gendered nature of caregiving responsibilities in the context of malaria highlights the need for gender-responsive interventions and support mechanisms. Recognizing and addressing the caregiving burden on women requires targeted approaches that take into account the unique challenges faced by women in malaria-endemic regions. This can involve providing access to support networks, childcare services, and income-generating opportunities that enable women to balance their caregiving responsibilities with other aspects of their lives.

Efforts to alleviate the caregiving burden on women can contribute to reducing gender inequalities and empowering women to actively participate in economic and educational pursuits. It is crucial to promote gender equality, challenge traditional gender roles, and create an enabling environment that supports women's empowerment and their ability to fulfill their caregiving responsibilities while pursuing their own goals.

6.2.3 Access to healthcare:

Access to healthcare is a critical factor in addressing malaria in West Africa, and gender disparities can hinder women's ability to seek timely diagnosis and treatment for the disease. Kilama et al. (2014) highlight that sociocultural norms, economic constraints, and limited decision-making power can restrict women's agency in accessing healthcare services for themselves and their families.

Sociocultural norms and gender roles may limit women's mobility and decision-making power, making it difficult for them to prioritize their own health needs. Economic constraints, including financial barriers and lack of resources, can further impede women's access to healthcare. Women's lower socioeconomic status and limited control over household resources can limit their ability to seek timely and appropriate healthcare services for themselves and their families.

These gender disparities in healthcare access can have significant implications for malaria control and prevention efforts. When women face barriers in accessing healthcare, including malaria diagnosis and treatment services, it can lead to delays in seeking care, increased disease severity, and higher transmission rates within communities.

Addressing gender disparities in healthcare access requires multi-faceted approaches. It involves promoting gender equality, challenging discriminatory norms and practices, and enhancing women's empowerment and decision-making abilities. This includes improving women's access to healthcare services, providing information and education on malaria prevention and treatment, and ensuring that healthcare facilities are gender-sensitive and accessible.

Efforts to address gender disparities in healthcare access should also consider the importance of engaging men and communities in promoting women's health and addressing gender norms and barriers. Community-based interventions, community health workers, and targeted outreach programs can play a crucial role in reaching women and addressing their specific healthcare needs.

6.2.4 Socioeconomic implications:

Malaria's impact on women's health and productivity can have long-term economic consequences, perpetuating poverty and gender disparities. (Littrell et al., 2013).

Women's reduced productivity due to malaria-related illnesses and caregiving responsibilities can limit their economic empowerment and hinder overall socio-economic development. (Littrell et al., 2013).

Investing in gender-responsive interventions, including access to education, economic opportunities, and healthcare services, is crucial for addressing the gender dimensions of malaria and promoting women's empowerment.

Efforts to address the gender dimensions of malaria require a comprehensive approach that includes integrating gender perspectives into malaria control strategies, strengthening health systems to provide accessible and gender-responsive services, and promoting gender equality and women's empowerment.

By addressing the specific challenges faced by women and girls in malaria-endemic regions, such as improving access to reproductive health services, enhancing educational opportunities, and promoting economic empowerment, it is possible to reduce the gender disparities associated with malaria and contribute to sustainable development.

6.3 Impact on social cohesion and community development

Malaria has a significant impact on social cohesion and community development in malaria-endemic regions. The following analysis explores the effects of malaria on social cohesion and community development, highlighting the challenges faced and potential solutions:

Disruption of social cohesion:

Malaria-related illnesses and deaths can have a significant impact on social cohesion within communities. As families and communities cope with the consequences of malaria, social networks may become disrupted and strained. Koenker et al. (2016) highlight that the burden of malaria can put a strain on social relationships and support systems, leading to increased stress and potential conflicts within communities.

The fear and stigma associated with malaria can further contribute to the disruption of social cohesion. Individuals and communities affected by malaria may face stigma and discrimination, leading to social exclusion and a breakdown of trust. This can create barriers to community engagement, hinder collective action in preventing and controlling malaria, and undermine community-based efforts for disease management (Ahorlu et al., 2019).

Moreover, the impact of malaria on social cohesion extends beyond individual families to the broader community level. The loss of productive community members due to malaria-related deaths can weaken social networks, reduce community resilience, and hinder collective efforts for development. Communities dealing with high malaria burden may experience increased stress, reduced cooperation, and limited resources for community-driven initiatives (Deressa et al., 2017).

Addressing the disruption of social cohesion caused by malaria requires a comprehensive approach that considers the social and cultural contexts of affected communities. Promoting community engagement, raising awareness about malaria prevention and control, and addressing stigma and discrimination associated with the disease are important steps towards rebuilding social cohesion. Strengthening community support systems, fostering dialogue, and promoting collaboration between community members, healthcare providers, and local authorities can help in creating a supportive environment for addressing the challenges posed by malaria.

6.3.1 Economic burden and poverty:

The economic burden of malaria is a significant contributor to poverty and social inequalities within communities. Malaria-related healthcare expenditures and productivity losses can push affected individuals and their families deeper into poverty. The costs associated with malaria treatment, including healthcare services, diagnostic tests, medications, and hospitalization, can impose a financial burden on households, particularly those with limited resources (Sachs & Malaney, 2002). These expenses can deplete already limited financial resources and hinder households' ability to meet their basic needs, invest in education, and participate in economic activities.

Furthermore, the economic burden of malaria extends beyond individual households to the broader community level. The costs associated with malaria treatment and prevention can strain healthcare systems and limit the allocation of resources for other essential services, such as education, infrastructure development, and community development initiatives. Ahorlu et al. (2019) highlight that the economic burden of malaria can undermine community efforts for progress and hinder overall development.

The economic burden of malaria contributes to a cycle of poverty and perpetuates social inequalities within communities. The financial hardships faced by affected individuals and households limit their opportunities for socio-economic advancement and reduce their resilience to future challenges. Moreover, the economic impact of malaria can exacerbate existing social inequalities, as vulnerable populations with limited resources are disproportionately affected (Sachs & Malaney, 2002). Addressing the economic burden of malaria requires a multi-sectoral approach that focuses on improving access to affordable healthcare services, implementing cost-effective prevention and control strategies, and promoting economic empowerment and poverty reduction initiatives.

6.3.2 Impact on community participation:

Malaria can have a significant impact on community participation and engagement in various development activities. The burden of malaria-related illnesses and the resulting reduced productivity can limit individuals' ability to actively participate in income-generating activities and community projects, thereby affecting community development efforts. Ahmed et al. (2013) highlight that malaria can impede community participation in key sectors such as education, agriculture, and local governance.

In the education sector, malaria-related absenteeism and the impact on cognitive development can disrupt children's regular attendance and hinder their academic performance. This can limit their educational opportunities and future prospects, as well as hinder community-wide efforts to improve literacy rates and educational outcomes. Additionally, the reduced productivity and increased healthcare burden associated with malaria can limit households' financial resources, making it difficult for them to invest in education-related expenses such as school fees, books, and uniforms.

In the agricultural sector, malaria-related illnesses can reduce the work capacity and productivity of farmers, leading to decreased agricultural output and lower incomes. This can hinder community-level efforts to improve food security, increase agricultural productivity, and alleviate poverty. The reduced participation of farmers in farming activities such as land preparation, planting, and harvesting can result in delayed or incomplete agricultural activities, affecting the overall agricultural productivity of the community.

Furthermore, the impact of malaria on community participation extends to local governance and community projects. The burden of malaria-related illnesses and the resulting economic hardships can limit individuals' time and resources available for engaging in community development initiatives. This can lead to reduced participation in local governance processes, community meetings, and decision-making, affecting the overall development and progress of the community.

Addressing the impact of malaria on community participation requires a comprehensive approach that includes effective malaria prevention and control strategies, access to quality healthcare services, and community empowerment initiatives. By reducing the burden of malaria and improving the overall health and well-being of community members, communities can enhance their capacity for active participation in various development activities. Promoting community engagement and ownership in malaria control efforts can also strengthen community resilience and contribute to sustainable development.

6.3.3 Strengthening social cohesion and community development:

Building community awareness and knowledge about malaria prevention, treatment, and control strategies is essential for fostering collective action and community engagement. (Ahorlu et al., 2019).

Strengthening local health systems, including access to quality healthcare and malaria interventions, can enhance community resilience and social cohesion. (Ahmed et al., 2013).

Empowering community leaders, women, and other key stakeholders to actively participate in malaria control programs and community development initiatives can contribute to sustainable progress. (Deressa et al., 2017).

Efforts to mitigate the impact of malaria on social cohesion and community development require multi-sectoral collaboration and community involvement. Integrating malaria control programs with broader community development initiatives, such as education, infrastructure, and income-generating projects, can foster resilience, social cohesion, and sustainable development.

Moreover, addressing the social determinants of malaria, such as poverty, inadequate healthcare, and limited access to education, is crucial for promoting social cohesion and community development in malaria-endemic regions. By focusing on community empowerment, equitable access to resources, and participatory decision-making processes, it is possible to build stronger and more resilient communities in the face of malaria.

Table 6: Impact of Malaria on Social Cohesion and Community Development

Aspect	Impact	Potential Solutions
Disruption of Social Cohesion	- Strained social networks and support systems due to malaria burden (Koenker et al., 2016). - Fear and stigma lead to social exclusion and breakdown of trust (Ahorlu et al., 2019). - Loss of productive community members weakens social networks and community resilience (Deressa et al., 2017).	- Promote community engagement and awareness about malaria prevention and control. - Address stigma and discrimination associated with the disease. - Strengthen community support systems and foster collaboration between stakeholders.
Economic Burden and Poverty	- Healthcare expenditures and productivity losses push households into poverty (Sachs & Malaney, 2002). - Strain on healthcare systems limits resources for development initiatives (Ahorlu et al., 2019). - Vulnerable populations are disproportionately affected (Sachs & Malaney, 2002).	- Improve access to affordable healthcare services. - Implement cost-effective prevention and control strategies. - Promote economic empowerment and poverty reduction initiatives.
Impact on Community Participation	- Absenteeism and reduced productivity disrupt education (Ahmed et al., 2013). - Reduced work capacity affects agricultural productivity and food security (Ahmed et al., 2013). - Economic hardships limit engagement in community projects (Ahmed et al., 2013).	- Enhance malaria prevention and control strategies. - Improve access to quality healthcare services. - Empower community leaders and key stakeholders to participate in malaria control and community development.
Strengthening Social Cohesion	- Foster community awareness about malaria prevention and control (Ahorlu et al., 2019). -	- Integrate malaria control with broader community development initiatives. -

THE IMPACT OF MALARIA ON THE SOCIAL-ECONOMIC DEVELOPMENT OF WEST AFRICA

Strengthen local health systems (Ahmed et al., 2013). - Empower community leaders and stakeholders (Deressa et al., 2017). Address social determinants of malaria, such as poverty and limited access to healthcare and education. - Promote community empowerment and participatory decision-making processes.

The table summarizes the impact of malaria on social cohesion and community development in malaria-endemic regions. It highlights disruptions in social networks, economic burdens, reduced community participation, and potential solutions, including community engagement and strengthening healthcare systems.

Chapter 7. Strategies for Malaria Control and Prevention

7.1 Overview of existing malaria control interventions

Malaria control interventions encompass a range of strategies aimed at reducing the transmission of the disease and mitigating its impact on public health. This section provides an overview of two key malaria control interventions: vector control and antimalarial drugs. The discussion is supported by relevant in-text citations:

7.1.1 Vector control:

7.1.1.1 Insecticide-treated bed nets (ITNs):

ITNs are a widely implemented intervention for malaria prevention. These nets are treated with insecticides that repel and kill mosquitoes, thereby reducing human-mosquito contact and preventing transmission. (Lengeler, 2004)

Indoor residual spraying (IRS): IRS involves the application of insecticides to the walls and ceilings of dwellings to kill mosquitoes that come into contact with the treated surfaces. IRS is effective in reducing malaria transmission in areas with susceptible mosquito populations. (Okumu et al., 2010)

7.1.1.2 Larval source management (LSM):

LSM INVOLVES TARGETING and eliminating mosquito breeding sites, such as stagnant water bodies, through drainage, larvicides, or environmental modifications. LSM can be effective in reducing mosquito populations and malaria transmission in specific settings. (Fillinger et al., 2009) [3]

7.1.2 Antimalarial drugs:

7.1.2.1 Artemisinin-based combination therapy (ACT):

ACT is the recommended first-line treatment for uncomplicated malaria caused by Plasmodium falciparum, the most prevalent malaria parasite. ACT combines an artemisinin derivative, which rapidly reduces the parasite load, with a partner drug that eliminates remaining parasites. (WHO, 2015)

7.1.2.2 Intermittent preventive treatment in pregnancy (IPTp):

IPTP INVOLVES ADMINISTERING antimalarial drugs to pregnant women, regardless of whether they are infected, to prevent malaria-related complications during pregnancy. Sulfadoxine-pyrimethamine is the recommended drug for IPTp. (WHO, 2012)

7.1.2.3 Seasonal malaria chemoprevention (SMC):

SMC INVOLVES ADMINISTERING antimalarial drugs to children in areas with highly seasonal malaria transmission. SMC is typically implemented during the peak transmission season to provide preventive treatment and reduce the incidence of malaria in this vulnerable population. (WHO, 2012).

These control interventions are implemented in combination to achieve maximum impact. The choice of interventions depends on the local epidemiology, vector species, drug resistance patterns, and available resources.

It is worth noting that the effectiveness of these interventions can be influenced by various factors, including insecticide resistance, community acceptance, healthcare access, and sustainable funding.

Therefore, a comprehensive and integrated approach, tailored to the local context, is essential for successful malaria control and elimination efforts.

7.2 Challenges and limitations of current approaches

While current malaria control interventions have made significant progress in reducing the burden of the disease, they still face several challenges and limitations. This section discusses some of the key challenges and limitations associated with current approaches to malaria control, supported by relevant in-text citations:

7.2.1 Insecticide resistance:

The emergence and spread of insecticide resistance among mosquito populations pose a major challenge to vector control interventions such as insecticide-treated bed nets and indoor residual spraying. Mosquitoes with resistance to commonly used insecticides may survive the insecticidal effects, reducing the effectiveness of these interventions. (Ranson et al., 2011)

Monitoring and managing insecticide resistance are crucial for sustaining the effectiveness of vector control interventions. However, limited resources, inadequate surveillance systems, and the development of multiple resistance mechanisms complicate these efforts. (Strode et al., 2014)

7.2.2 Drug resistance:

The emergence and spread of drug-resistant malaria parasites, particularly to artemisinin-based combination therapies (ACTs), pose a significant threat to effective treatment. Resistance to artemisinins has been reported in Southeast Asia, raising concerns about the potential spread to other regions. (Takala-Harrison & Laufer, 2015).

Delayed parasite clearance, reduced treatment efficacy, and increased treatment failure rates associated with drug resistance undermine the effectiveness of antimalarial drug interventions. Ongoing monitoring, surveillance, and development of alternative treatment options are essential to address this challenge. (WHO, 2019).

7.2.3 Access to interventions:

Limited access to malaria control interventions, including insecticide-treated bed nets, antimalarial drugs, and diagnostic tests, remains a major barrier in many malaria-endemic regions. Economic constraints, geographical remoteness, weak health systems, and inadequate distribution channels contribute to inequitable access. (WHO, 2019).

Disparities in access to interventions can further exacerbate malaria burden among vulnerable populations, such as marginalized communities, migrants, and refugees. Ensuring equitable access to interventions is crucial for effective malaria control and elimination. (WHO, 2019).

7.2.4 Behavioral and cultural factors:

Malaria control interventions heavily rely on community engagement and individual behavior change. However, behavioral factors, such as inconsistent use of bed nets or delays in seeking treatment, can hinder the effectiveness of interventions. Cultural beliefs, misconceptions, and stigma associated with malaria may also impact the uptake and acceptance of control measures. (Chukwuocha et al., 2015).

Tailoring interventions to local contexts, addressing cultural and social factors, and fostering community participation and ownership are essential for sustainable behavior change and improved intervention effectiveness. (Deressa et al., 2017).

Addressing these challenges requires a multi-faceted approach, including the development of new insecticides and antimalarial drugs, strengthening surveillance systems for resistance monitoring, improving access to interventions through innovative delivery strategies, and promoting community engagement and behavior change. Additionally, sustained financial and political commitments at global, regional, and national levels are vital to overcoming these challenges and advancing malaria control efforts.

7.3 Examination of innovative strategies and technologies for malaria control in West Africa

In West Africa, where malaria remains a significant public health concern, several innovative strategies and technologies are being explored and implemented to enhance malaria control efforts. The following examination highlights some of these innovative approaches, supported by relevant in-text citations:

7.3.1 Long-lasting insecticidal nets (LLINs):

LLINs, which are insecticide-treated bed nets designed to retain their efficacy for an extended period, have been widely adopted as a key malaria control intervention. They have shown effectiveness in reducing malaria transmission and morbidity in West Africa. (Alout et al., 2014)

Innovative techniques such as piperonyl butoxide (PBO)-based LLINs, which enhance the insecticidal effectiveness against insecticide-resistant mosquitoes, have been developed and tested in West Africa. These nets have demonstrated improved performance in areas with high insecticide resistance. (Pennetier et al., 2013).

7.3.2 Indoor residual spraying (IRS):

Innovative formulations and strategies for indoor residual spraying have been explored to improve the effectiveness and sustainability of this intervention. For example, new insecticide formulations, such as microencapsulated and water-dispersible formulations, have been developed and tested in West Africa to enhance residual insecticidal activity and mitigate insecticide resistance. (Aïkpon et al., 2014).

Targeted IRS campaigns that focus on high-transmission areas or specific populations at higher risk, such as pregnant women and children, have shown promise in maximizing the impact of IRS interventions. (Koudou et al., 2010).

7.3.3 Larval source management (LSM):

Innovative approaches to larval source management, such as the use of biological control agents and environmental management techniques, are being explored in West Africa. Biological control involves introducing mosquito predators or pathogens to reduce mosquito populations, while environmental management focuses on modifying or eliminating mosquito breeding sites. These approaches have shown potential in reducing vector populations and malaria transmission. (Fillinger et al., 2009).

7.3.4 Community-based interventions:

Community-based interventions, including community health workers and community-led surveillance, have been implemented to enhance malaria control in West Africa. By engaging and empowering communities, these interventions aim to improve case management, promote behavior change, and strengthen surveillance and reporting systems. (WHO, 2019) [6]

Mobile health technologies, such as text messaging and mobile applications, are being utilized to support community-based interventions, including health education, case management, and reporting of malaria cases. These technologies have shown promise in enhancing communication, data collection, and surveillance in resource-limited settings. (L'Engle et al., 2016).

These innovative strategies and technologies, when integrated into comprehensive malaria control programs, have the potential to contribute to the reduction of malaria transmission and morbidity in West Africa. However, it is crucial to ensure that these approaches are contextually appropriate, sustainable, and tailored to the local epidemiological and social factors.

Further research, evaluation, and collaboration between researchers, policymakers, and communities are needed to refine and scale up these innovative strategies and technologies, with the ultimate goal of achieving sustainable malaria control and elimination in West Africa.

Chapter 8. The Role of International Partnerships and Global Initiatives

8.1 Analysis of international efforts to combat malaria in West Africa

International efforts to combat malaria in West Africa have been significant, aiming to reduce the burden of the disease, strengthen health systems, and promote sustainable malaria control and elimination. The following analysis explores key international initiatives and interventions implemented in West Africa, highlighting their contributions and challenges:

8.1.1 Global Fund to Fight AIDS, Tuberculosis and Malaria:

The Global Fund has played a crucial role in supporting malaria control efforts in West Africa through financing and coordinating interventions. It has provided funding for the procurement of insecticide-treated bed nets, antimalarial drugs, diagnostics, and capacity-building activities. (Global Fund, n.d.)

Challenges faced include sustaining financial support, ensuring efficient use of funds, strengthening health systems, and addressing barriers to access in remote and underserved areas.

8.1.2 President's Malaria Initiative (PMI):

PMI, led by the United States Agency for International Development (USAID) in collaboration with other partners, has been instrumental in supporting malaria control and elimination efforts in West Africa. It focuses on providing technical assistance, capacity building, and resources for interventions such as bed net distribution, indoor residual spraying, and case management. (PMI, n.d.).

Challenges include the need for sustained funding, aligning interventions with national strategies, addressing insecticide and drug resistance, and ensuring coordination among partners.

8.1.3 Roll Back Malaria (RBM) Partnership:

RBM is a global partnership that aims to coordinate and advocate for malaria control and elimination efforts. It supports countries in West Africa through strategic guidance, knowledge sharing, and resource mobilization. RBM promotes the implementation of integrated malaria control strategies, including vector control, case management, and advocacy for political commitment. (RBM Partnership, n.d.).

Challenges include aligning diverse partners' priorities, maintaining political commitment, fostering collaboration among sectors, and ensuring sustained funding and resources.

8.1.4 Research and Innovation:

International organizations and research institutions collaborate with West African countries to conduct research on malaria prevention, treatment, and control. This includes studies on insecticide and drug resistance, vector behavior, diagnostics, and innovative interventions. Research findings contribute to evidence-based policy and programmatic decisions. (WHO, 2019).

Challenges include translating research findings into practical interventions, ensuring research relevance to local contexts, and building local research capacity.

These international efforts have contributed to significant progress in malaria control in West Africa. However, challenges persist, including the need for sustained funding, strengthening health systems, addressing insecticide and drug resistance, promoting community engagement, and ensuring equitable access to interventions. Collaboration among international partners, national governments, civil society, and communities is crucial to overcome these challenges and achieve sustained malaria control and elimination in the region.

Table 7 International Efforts to Combat Malaria in West Africa

Initiative	Description	Contributions	Challenges
Global Fund to Fight AIDS, Tuberculosis, and Malaria	The Global Fund provides financing and coordination of interventions in West Africa, including procurement of bed nets, drugs, diagnostics, and capacity-building activities. (Global Fund, n.d.)	Financial support, coordination of interventions	Sustaining financial support, efficient use of funds, strengthening health systems, addressing barriers to access in remote and underserved areas
President's Malaria Initiative (PMI)	Led by USAID, PMI supports malaria control and elimination efforts in West Africa through technical assistance, capacity building, and resources for interventions such as bed nets, indoor spraying, and case management. (PMI, n.d.)	Technical assistance, capacity building, resources for interventions	Sustained funding, alignment with national strategies, insecticide and drug resistance, coordination among partners
Roll Back Malaria (RBM) Partnership	RBM coordinates and advocates for malaria control and elimination in West Africa, providing strategic guidance, knowledge sharing, and resource mobilization. It promotes integrated control strategies and political commitment. (RBM Partnership, n.d.)	Strategic guidance, resource mobilization, knowledge sharing	Partner alignment, political commitment, collaboration among sectors, sustained funding and resources
Research and Innovation	International organizations and research institutions collaborate with West African countries to conduct research on malaria	Research on prevention, treatment, control	Translation of research findings, relevance to local contexts, local

THE IMPACT OF MALARIA ON THE SOCIAL-ECONOMIC DEVELOPMENT OF WEST AFRICA

prevention, treatment, and control. Research findings contribute to evidence-based decision-making. (WHO, 2019)

research capacity

Description: The table summarizes key international initiatives to combat malaria in West Africa, including the Global Fund to Fight AIDS, Tuberculosis, and Malaria; the President's Malaria Initiative (PMI); the Roll Back Malaria (RBM) Partnership; and research and innovation.

8.2 Examination of key initiatives

8.2.1 Roll Back Malaria Partnership:

The Roll Back Malaria (RBM) Partnership is a global initiative established in 1998 to coordinate and accelerate malaria control efforts worldwide. It brings together various stakeholders, including governments, international organizations, civil society, and the private sector, to work collaboratively towards malaria control and elimination. The RBM Partnership focuses on four key areas:

8.2.1.1 Advocacy and resource mobilization:

RBM ADVOCATES FOR INCREASED political commitment and resources to support malaria control programs. It raises awareness about the impact of malaria and the need for sustained investment, encouraging governments and donors to prioritize malaria control in their agendas.

8.2.1.2 Technical guidance and support:

THE RBM PARTNERSHIP provides technical guidance to countries, helping them develop and implement effective malaria control strategies. It promotes the adoption of evidence-based interventions, such as vector control, case management, and preventive therapies, and supports countries in strengthening their health systems.

8.2.1.3 Monitoring and evaluation:

RBM FACILITATES MONITORING and evaluation of malaria control programs to track progress, assess impact, and identify gaps. It promotes the use of standardized indicators and data collection methods, enabling countries to measure their malaria burden and evaluate the effectiveness of interventions.

8.2.1.4 Partnerships and collaboration:

162

RBM FOSTERS PARTNERSHIPS among stakeholders involved in malaria control, encouraging collaboration and knowledge sharing. It promotes coordination among international organizations, governments, civil society, and communities to ensure a comprehensive and integrated approach to malaria control.

8.2.2 Global Fund to Fight AIDS, Tuberculosis, and Malaria:

The Global Fund is a financing mechanism established in 2002 to mobilize resources and support the fight against HIV/AIDS, tuberculosis, and malaria. It provides financial support to countries to implement prevention, treatment, and control interventions. Key features of the Global Fund's approach include:

8.2.2.1 Country ownership:

THE GLOBAL FUND EMPHASIZES country ownership, working closely with national governments and partners to develop and implement malaria control programs tailored to each country's context. This approach ensures that interventions are aligned with national strategies and priorities.

8.2.2.2 Funding and grants:

THE GLOBAL FUND MOBILIZES financial resources from governments, private sector partners, and other donors and channels them to eligible countries through grant mechanisms. These grants support a range of activities, including the procurement of bed nets, antimalarial drugs, diagnostics, strengthening health systems, and capacity building.

8.2.2.3 Technical support and capacity building:

IN ADDITION TO FINANCIAL support, the Global Fund provides technical assistance and capacity building to countries. This support aims to strengthen health systems, enhance program management and implementation, and improve monitoring and evaluation practices.

8.2.2.4 Performance-based funding:

THE GLOBAL FUND ADOPTS a performance-based funding approach, linking the disbursement of funds to countries' achievement of predetermined targets and outcomes. This incentivizes countries to demonstrate results and accountability in their malaria control efforts.

Both the Roll Back Malaria Partnership and the Global Fund have played instrumental roles in driving progress in malaria control and elimination in West Africa. Their efforts have contributed to increased funding, improved access to interventions, strengthened health systems, and enhanced coordination among stakeholders. However, challenges remain, such as sustaining financial support, addressing emerging issues like insecticide and drug resistance, and ensuring equitable access to interventions for vulnerable populations. Continued collaboration and commitment from these initiatives, along with national governments and other stakeholders, are crucial to overcoming these challenges and achieving sustained malaria control in the region.

8.3 The importance of collaboration between governments, NGOs, and the private sector

8.3.1 Collaborations

Collaboration between governments, non-governmental organizations (NGOs), and the private sector is of paramount importance in the fight against malaria in West Africa. Each sector brings unique strengths and resources to the table, and working together synergistically can lead to more effective and sustainable malaria control efforts. The following points highlight the significance of collaboration:

8.3.1.1 Resource mobilization:

GOVERNMENTS, NGOS, and the private sector all play a crucial role in mobilizing resources for malaria control. Governments can allocate funds and create policies that prioritize malaria control in national agendas. NGOs can leverage their networks and engage in fundraising efforts to support malaria programs. The private sector can contribute financial resources, expertise, and innovative technologies for the development and implementation of interventions.

8.3.1.2 Knowledge and expertise sharing:

COLLABORATION ALLOWS for the sharing of knowledge, experiences, and best practices among different sectors. Governments can provide valuable insights into the local context, epidemiology, and health systems, while NGOs can contribute their field-level experience and technical expertise. The private sector can bring innovative ideas and technologies based on their research and development efforts. This exchange of knowledge leads to informed decision-making and more effective implementation strategies.

8.3.1.3 Program implementation and service delivery:

COLLABORATION ENABLES coordinated efforts in program implementation and service delivery. Governments can provide the necessary infrastructure, logistics, and regulatory frameworks to support malaria control interventions. NGOs can assist in community engagement, capacity building, and frontline service delivery. The private sector can contribute by supporting the production, distribution, and delivery of essential tools and commodities such as bed nets, diagnostics, and antimalarial drugs.

8.3.1.4 Advocacy and policy development:

COLLABORATION BETWEEN sectors amplifies advocacy efforts for malaria control. Governments can advocate for increased political commitment and resource allocation at the national and international levels. NGOs can engage in advocacy campaigns, raise public awareness, and advocate for policy changes that promote malaria control. The private sector can leverage its influence to advocate for corporate social responsibility and support policy development that aligns with malaria control goals.

8.3.1.5 Innovation and technology:

COLLABORATION BETWEEN sectors facilitates innovation and the development of new technologies for malaria control. Governments can provide a regulatory framework that fosters innovation and facilitates the introduction of new interventions. NGOs can collaborate with researchers and implement pilot projects to test innovative approaches. The private sector, with its research and development capabilities, can contribute by developing new tools, diagnostics, and insecticides.

8.3.1.6 Sustainable partnerships:

COLLABORATION FOSTERS long-term partnerships that are essential for sustained malaria control efforts. Governments, NGOs, and the private sector can establish formal partnerships that outline shared objectives, responsibilities, and mechanisms for monitoring and evaluation. Such partnerships ensure continuity, resource mobilization, and collective accountability in the fight against malaria.

While collaboration between governments, NGOs, and the private sector offers numerous benefits, challenges also exist. These include aligning priorities and strategies, ensuring transparency, addressing power dynamics, and maintaining sustained engagement and commitment. Effective collaboration requires strong leadership, clear communication channels, shared goals, and mutual trust among all stakeholders.

In conclusion, collaboration between governments, NGOs, and the private sector is vital for the success of malaria control efforts in West Africa. By leveraging their respective strengths, resources, and expertise, these sectors can contribute to the development and implementation of comprehensive, sustainable, and impactful strategies that aim to reduce the burden of malaria and ultimately eliminate the disease.

Chapter 9. Case Studies: Successful Malaria Control Programs in West Africa

9.1 Some countries or regions that have made significant progress in malaria control

Several countries and regions in West Africa have made significant progress in malaria control, demonstrating that with the right interventions and sustained efforts, malaria burden can be reduced. The following highlight countries and regions that have achieved notable success:

9.1.1 Senegal:

Senegal has been recognized as a success story in malaria control. Through strong political commitment, effective partnerships, and innovative strategies, the country has made remarkable progress in reducing malaria transmission and burden. Senegal has implemented a comprehensive approach that includes increased access to insecticide-treated bed nets, indoor residual spraying, effective case management, and community engagement. As a result, malaria-related mortality and morbidity have significantly declined in the country.

9.1.2 The Gambia:

The Gambia has made remarkable strides in malaria control. The country has implemented a combination of interventions, including widespread distribution of insecticide-treated bed nets, indoor residual spraying, and effective case management. The Gambia has also prioritized community involvement and engagement, empowering communities to take ownership of malaria control activities. These efforts have led to a substantial reduction in malaria cases and related deaths.

9.1.3 Zanzibar (Tanzania):

The Zanzibar archipelago, a region of Tanzania, has achieved significant progress in malaria control and is on the path towards malaria elimination. Zanzibar has implemented a comprehensive approach that includes distribution of insecticide-treated bed nets, indoor residual spraying, and timely and effective treatment of malaria cases. The region has also adopted innovative strategies such as community-based surveillance and response systems, as well as reactive case detection. As a result, malaria transmission has been dramatically reduced, and the region is now focused on sustaining these achievements and working towards malaria elimination.

Liberia is one of the countries that have made significant progress in malaria control. In recent years, Liberia has implemented various interventions and strategies to combat malaria and reduce its burden. These efforts have resulted in notable achievements in malaria control and prevention.

One of the key initiatives in Liberia's malaria control efforts is the distribution of insecticide-treated bed nets (ITNs) to vulnerable populations. The government, in collaboration with international partners and non-governmental organizations, has conducted mass distribution campaigns to increase the coverage of ITNs across the country. This has helped to protect individuals from mosquito bites and reduce malaria transmission.

Liberia has also focused on improving access to accurate malaria diagnosis and effective treatment. Rapid diagnostic tests (RDTs) have been widely deployed in healthcare facilities, enabling prompt and accurate diagnosis of malaria cases. This has facilitated targeted treatment and reduced the unnecessary use of antimalarial drugs.

Furthermore, Liberia has implemented indoor residual spraying (IRS) in areas with high malaria transmission. IRS involves the application of insecticides to the walls of houses, killing mosquitoes and reducing their population. This intervention has contributed to the reduction of malaria transmission in targeted areas.

In addition to these specific interventions, Liberia has made efforts to strengthen its healthcare system and enhance the capacity of healthcare workers in malaria diagnosis, treatment, and surveillance. This includes training programs, provision of essential malaria drugs and supplies, and the establishment of monitoring and evaluation systems to track progress and identify areas for improvement.

These comprehensive malaria control efforts in Liberia have resulted in a significant decline in malaria cases and deaths. According to the World Health Organization (WHO), malaria cases in Liberia decreased by over 50% between 2015 and 2019. This progress is a testament to the commitment of the Liberian government, the collaboration with international partners, and the engagement of local communities in malaria control activities.

However, despite the progress made, malaria remains a public health challenge in Liberia, particularly during the peak transmission season. Continued efforts are needed to sustain and further strengthen malaria control interventions, improve access to healthcare services, and address any emerging challenges such as insecticide resistance and changes in malaria epidemiology.

9.1.5 São Tomé and Príncipe:

São Tomé and Príncipe, a small island nation off the western coast of Central Africa, has made significant progress in malaria control. The country has implemented successful interventions such as widespread distribution of insecticide-treated bed nets, improved access to diagnostic testing, and effective treatment of malaria cases. São Tomé and Príncipe has also prioritized cross-sectoral collaboration and community involvement. These efforts have led to a substantial decrease in malaria incidence and mortality.

9.1.6 Eswatini (formerly Swaziland):

Eswatini has made remarkable progress in malaria control and is working towards malaria elimination. The country has implemented a combination of interventions, including widespread distribution of insecticide-treated bed nets, indoor residual spraying, and effective case management. Eswatini has also prioritized cross-border collaboration with neighboring countries to address importation of malaria cases. These efforts have led to a significant reduction in malaria burden, with a goal of achieving malaria elimination in the near future.

These examples highlight that significant progress in malaria control is achievable through a comprehensive and integrated approach, strong political commitment, effective partnerships, community engagement, and innovative strategies. These success stories provide valuable lessons and inspiration for other countries and regions in West Africa, emphasizing the importance of tailored approaches and sustained efforts in the fight against malaria.

9.2 Analysis of the factors contributing to their success

The success of countries and regions in malaria control can be attributed to several key factors. Understanding these factors is crucial for replicating and adapting successful strategies in other contexts. The following are some key factors contributing to the success of countries and regions in malaria control:

9.2.1 Strong political commitment:

Strong political commitment is indeed a critical factor in the success of malaria control efforts. Countries and regions that have made significant progress in malaria control have demonstrated a clear and unwavering commitment at the highest levels of government. This commitment is evident through the prioritization of malaria on national agendas, the allocation of sufficient resources, and the implementation of supportive policies.

An example of strong political commitment can be seen in Ethiopia. The Ethiopian government has shown a strong commitment to malaria control, leading to remarkable progress in reducing the burden of the disease. The government has developed a comprehensive national malaria control program and integrated it into the country's overall health system. The program focuses on key interventions such as the distribution of insecticide-treated bed nets, indoor residual spraying, and prompt diagnosis and treatment of malaria cases (Ethiopian Public Health Institute, 2020).

Ethiopia's political commitment to malaria control is reflected in its allocation of resources. The government has increased domestic funding for malaria control activities and secured support from international partners, including the Global Fund to Fight AIDS, Tuberculosis, and Malaria. These resources have been used to strengthen healthcare infrastructure, improve access to diagnostic tools and antimalarial drugs, and expand community-based malaria prevention and treatment programs (Ethiopian Public Health Institute, 2020).

Furthermore, Ethiopia has implemented policies that support effective malaria control interventions. The government has adopted evidence-based strategies and guidelines for malaria prevention, diagnosis, and treatment, aligning them with global best practices. The policies emphasize the importance of community engagement, integrated health services, and collaboration between different sectors, such as health, agriculture, and education (Ethiopian Public Health Institute, 2020).

This strong political commitment and comprehensive approach to malaria control in Ethiopia have yielded significant results. The country has achieved a substantial reduction in malaria cases and deaths over the years. According to the World Health Organization (WHO), Ethiopia recorded a 72% decrease in malaria cases and a 75% decrease in malaria-related deaths between 2015 and 2019 (WHO, 2020).

The example of Ethiopia highlights the importance of strong political commitment in driving successful malaria control efforts. When governments prioritize malaria, allocate adequate resources, and implement supportive policies, it creates an enabling environment for effective interventions and sustained progress in malaria control.

9.2.2 Comprehensive approach:

A comprehensive approach to malaria control has indeed been instrumental in the success of countries and regions in reducing the burden of the disease. By implementing a range of interventions that target different stages of the malaria transmission cycle, these areas have achieved significant progress in malaria control.

One example of a country that has adopted a comprehensive approach is Rwanda. The Rwandan government has implemented a multi-faceted malaria control strategy that includes the distribution of insecticide-treated bed nets, indoor residual spraying, and effective case management (Republic of Rwanda Ministry of Health, 2019). The distribution of bed nets aims to protect individuals from mosquito bites, while indoor residual spraying targets the reduction of mosquito populations by spraying insecticides on the walls of houses (Republic of Rwanda Ministry of Health, 2019). These interventions work together to prevent malaria transmission and reduce the number of cases.

Rwanda has also prioritized effective case management by ensuring prompt diagnosis and treatment of malaria cases. The country has implemented the use of rapid diagnostic tests to accurately diagnose malaria and has adopted artemisinin-based combination therapies (ACTs) as the first-line treatment for uncomplicated malaria (Republic of Rwanda Ministry of Health, 2019). These strategies ensure that individuals infected with malaria receive timely and appropriate treatment, which helps to reduce the severity of the disease and prevent complications.

In addition to these interventions, Rwanda emphasizes community engagement in its malaria control efforts. The government actively involves communities in malaria prevention and control activities through health education, community mobilization, and the establishment of community health workers (Republic of Rwanda Ministry of Health, 2019). This approach helps to raise awareness about malaria prevention measures, encourages community participation, and strengthens the overall impact of malaria control interventions.

Through this comprehensive approach, Rwanda has achieved significant progress in malaria control. According to the World Health Organization (WHO), between 2010 and 2019, Rwanda recorded a 78% decrease in malaria cases and a 79% decrease in malaria-related deaths (WHO, 2020). These achievements demonstrate the effectiveness of a comprehensive approach in reducing the burden of malaria.

The example of Rwanda highlights the importance of implementing a combination of interventions and engaging communities in malaria control efforts. By targeting multiple aspects of the malaria transmission cycle and involving various stakeholders, countries and regions can maximize the impact of their malaria control programs and make substantial progress in reducing the burden of the disease.

9.2.3 Collaboration and partnerships:

Collaboration and partnerships play a crucial role in successful malaria control efforts, bringing together diverse stakeholders and leveraging their collective strengths. Through collaboration, countries and regions have been able to make significant progress in malaria control by pooling resources, sharing expertise, and implementing coordinated interventions.

One example of successful collaboration is the partnership between Ghana and the Global Fund to Fight AIDS, Tuberculosis, and Malaria. Ghana has established strong partnerships with the Global Fund and other international organizations to strengthen its malaria control efforts. The collaboration has facilitated the mobilization of financial resources, procurement of essential commodities, and technical support for malaria prevention and treatment programs (Global Fund, 2020). By working together, Ghana and its partners have been able to scale up interventions, improve access to quality healthcare services, and reduce the burden of malaria in the country.

Another example is the Roll Back Malaria (RBM) Partnership, which brings together governments, non-governmental organizations, research institutions, and other stakeholders to coordinate malaria control efforts globally. The RBM Partnership promotes collaboration and partnership at the national and international levels, providing a platform for knowledge exchange, resource mobilization, and advocacy for malaria control (Roll Back Malaria Partnership, n.d.). Through this partnership, countries have been able to access technical expertise, funding opportunities, and best practices in malaria control, leading to improved program implementation and better health outcomes.

Furthermore, community engagement and partnerships with local organizations have been key to successful malaria control in many regions. For instance, in Senegal, the Malaria Research and Training Center (MRTC) collaborates with local communities, community-based organizations, and health authorities to implement malaria control interventions (Malaria Research and Training Center, n.d.). These partnerships enable community participation, local ownership, and the development of context-specific strategies for malaria control.

Collaboration and partnerships have been instrumental in achieving progress in malaria control by promoting synergy, avoiding duplication of efforts, and maximizing the impact of interventions. By working together, stakeholders can leverage their respective strengths, share resources, and develop innovative approaches tailored to the specific needs and challenges of malaria-endemic regions.

Through collaborative efforts, countries and regions have achieved notable results. For example, in Senegal, malaria cases decreased by 65% between 2010 and 2019, and malaria-related deaths declined by 73% during the same period (WHO, 2020). These achievements are a testament to the power of collaboration in malaria control.

Overall, collaboration and partnerships are essential components of successful malaria control efforts. By bringing together diverse stakeholders, fostering cooperation, and harnessing collective expertise, countries and regions can strengthen their malaria control programs and make significant progress in reducing the burden of the disease.

9.2.4 Community involvement and engagement:

Community involvement and engagement are indeed crucial elements of successful malaria control efforts. When communities are actively engaged in decision-making, implementation, and monitoring of malaria control activities, it enhances the effectiveness and sustainability of interventions. Communities play a vital role in advocating for malaria control, mobilizing resources, and ensuring the uptake of preventive measures. Several examples highlight the importance of community involvement in malaria control.

In Ghana, the National Malaria Control Program (NMCP) has implemented community-based initiatives to engage local communities in malaria control. Through community health workers and community leaders, the NMCP has educated community members about malaria prevention, distributed bed nets, and promoted the use of insecticide-treated bed nets (ITNs) (National Malaria Control Program, n.d.). This community-driven approach has not only increased the accessibility and utilization of bed nets but also empowered communities to take ownership of malaria control efforts.

In Nigeria, the Community Directed Intervention (CDI) approach has been successfully employed to engage communities in malaria control. The CDI approach involves training community volunteers who play a vital role in the distribution of ITNs, administration of antimalarial drugs, and community mobilization for behavior change (Uzochukwu et al., 2011). By involving community members in decision-making and implementation, the CDI approach ensures that interventions are culturally appropriate and tailored to the specific needs of the community.

The involvement of communities in vector control efforts, such as indoor residual spraying (IRS) and larval source management (LSM), has also proven effective in malaria control. In Burkina Faso, community participation in IRS has been achieved through community-led organizations responsible for implementing and monitoring IRS activities (Gonçalves et al., 2016). This participatory approach has not only increased the coverage of IRS but also empowered communities to take ownership of their health.

Furthermore, community engagement is essential for promoting behavior change and sustaining malaria control interventions. In Tanzania, community dialogues and social marketing campaigns have been employed to increase community awareness and promote the use of ITNs (Koenker et al., 2015). These community-driven initiatives have resulted in improved ITN usage and contributed to the reduction of malaria transmission.

Community involvement and engagement in malaria control activities foster a sense of ownership, increase compliance with interventions, and promote sustainable behavior change. By actively involving community members, their knowledge, experiences, and perspectives are integrated into program design and implementation. This approach ensures that interventions are culturally appropriate, accepted, and effectively address the specific challenges faced by each community.

9.2.5 Evidence-based decision-making:

Community involvement and engagement are indeed crucial elements of successful malaria control efforts. When communities are actively engaged in decision-making, implementation, and monitoring of malaria control activities, it enhances the effectiveness and sustainability of interventions. Communities play a vital role in advocating for malaria control, mobilizing resources, and ensuring the uptake of preventive measures. Several examples highlight the importance of community involvement in malaria control.

In Ghana, the National Malaria Control Program (NMCP) has implemented community-based initiatives to engage local communities in malaria control. Through community health workers and community leaders, the NMCP has educated community members about malaria prevention, distributed bed nets, and promoted the use of insecticide-treated bed nets (ITNs) (National Malaria Control Program, n.d.). This community-driven approach has not only increased the accessibility and utilization of bed nets but also empowered communities to take ownership of malaria control efforts.

In Nigeria, the Community Directed Intervention (CDI) approach has been successfully employed to engage communities in malaria control. The CDI approach involves training community volunteers who play a vital role in the distribution of ITNs, administration of antimalarial drugs, and community mobilization for behavior change (Uzochukwu et al., 2011). By involving community members in decision-making and implementation, the CDI approach ensures that interventions are culturally appropriate and tailored to the specific needs of the community.

The involvement of communities in vector control efforts, such as indoor residual spraying (IRS) and larval source management (LSM), has also proven effective in malaria control. In Burkina Faso, community participation in IRS has been achieved through community-led organizations responsible for implementing and monitoring IRS activities (Gonçalves et al., 2016). This participatory approach has not only increased the coverage of IRS but also empowered communities to take ownership of their health.

Furthermore, community engagement is essential for promoting behavior change and sustaining malaria control interventions. In Tanzania, community dialogues and social marketing campaigns have been employed to increase community awareness and promote the use of ITNs (Koenker et al., 2015). These community-driven initiatives have resulted in improved ITN usage and contributed to the reduction of malaria transmission.

Community involvement and engagement in malaria control activities foster a sense of ownership, increase compliance with interventions, and promote sustainable behavior change. By actively involving community members, their knowledge, experiences, and perspectives are integrated into program design and implementation. This approach ensures that interventions are culturally appropriate, accepted, and effectively address the specific challenges faced by each community.

9.2.6 Adaptability and innovation:

Adaptability and innovation are key factors in successful malaria control efforts. Countries and regions that have made significant progress in malaria control demonstrate the ability to adapt their strategies and embrace innovative approaches to address emerging challenges. They continuously evaluate the effectiveness of interventions and make necessary adjustments to optimize outcomes. Examples of adaptability and innovation in malaria control can be found in various contexts.

In Zambia, the National Malaria Elimination Program (NMEP) has embraced innovative approaches to malaria control. They have implemented a mobile phone-based reporting system called the District Health Information System (DHIS2) to enhance surveillance and data collection (Chanda et al., 2012). This technology allows for real-time reporting of malaria cases, facilitating timely decision-making and targeted interventions. The use of DHIS2 has improved the efficiency and accuracy of data collection, enabling the NMEP to track the progress of malaria control efforts and identify areas requiring intervention.

Another example of adaptability and innovation can be seen in the use of new vector control techniques. In some regions, the deployment of insecticide-treated eave curtains (ITECs) has been explored as an alternative or complementary intervention to bed nets and indoor residual spraying (IRS). ITECs are specially designed curtains that release insecticides, targeting mosquitoes as they attempt to enter houses through the eaves (Koenker et al., 2017). This approach has shown promising results in reducing malaria transmission in areas where mosquitoes predominantly enter houses through eaves rather than windows or doors.

In addition, innovative community engagement strategies have been employed to promote behavior change and sustain malaria control efforts. In Nigeria, the Malaria Consortium implemented the Support to National Malaria Program (SuNMaP) project, which involved the use of theater performances, community dialogues, and peer education to engage communities and deliver key malaria prevention messages (Malaria Consortium, 2013). These innovative approaches aimed to capture the attention of community members, improve knowledge, and promote positive behavioral practices for malaria prevention.

By embracing adaptability and innovation, successful countries and regions in malaria control can effectively respond to emerging challenges, improve program efficiency, and optimize resource utilization. They explore new technologies, approaches, and strategies to enhance surveillance, vector control, and community engagement. These innovative efforts contribute to the overall effectiveness and sustainability of malaria control interventions, ultimately leading to improved outcomes in reducing the burden of malaria.

Regional collaboration and cross-border initiatives:

Countries and regions have also achieved success through regional collaboration and cross-border initiatives. Malaria knows no boundaries, and cooperation between neighboring countries is crucial for addressing cross-border malaria transmission. Sharing information, harmonizing strategies, and coordinating efforts contribute to reducing importation of malaria cases and maintaining control in border areas.

It is important to note that the success factors may vary depending on the context and specific challenges faced by each country or region. Tailoring interventions to the local epidemiology, considering socio-cultural factors, and ensuring health system strengthening are also important components of successful malaria control efforts.

By analyzing these factors, countries and regions can draw insights and lessons from successful examples, adapt strategies to their own context, and work towards sustainable malaria control and elimination

Table 8: Factors Contributing to the Success of Malaria Control in West Africa

Factors	Examples
Strong political commitment	Ethiopia: Comprehensive national malaria control program, increased domestic funding, supportive policies (Ethiopian Public Health Institute, 2020)
Comprehensive approach	Rwanda: Bed net distribution, indoor residual spraying, effective case management (Republic of Rwanda Ministry of Health, 2019)
Collaboration and partnerships	Ghana: Collaboration with the Global Fund for financial resources and technical support (Global Fund, 2020)
Community involvement and engagement	Ghana: Community-based initiatives, involvement of community health workers (National Malaria Control Program, n.d.)
Adaptability and innovation	Zambia: Use of mobile phone-based reporting system (Chanda et al., 2012)
Regional collaboration and cross-border initiatives	Cross-border cooperation to address importation and transmission of malaria cases

The table presents key factors contributing to the success of malaria control in West Africa. These factors include strong political commitment, a comprehensive approach encompassing multiple interventions, collaboration and partnerships, community involvement and engagement, adaptability and innovation, and regional collaboration.

9.3 Lessons learned and implications for future interventions

The success stories in malaria control from various countries and regions in West Africa provide valuable lessons and insights that can inform future interventions. The following are some key lessons learned and implications for future malaria control interventions:

9.3.1 Tailored approaches:

One size does not fit all when it comes to malaria control. Successful interventions have demonstrated the importance of tailoring strategies to the local context, taking into account factors such as epidemiology, socio-cultural norms, and health system capacity. Future interventions should prioritize context-specific approaches that address the unique challenges and opportunities of each region or country.

9.3.2 Comprehensive and integrated interventions:

The success of malaria control efforts lies in implementing a comprehensive and integrated approach. Combining multiple interventions, such as vector control, case management, community engagement, and surveillance, creates synergistic effects and maximizes impact. Future interventions should prioritize comprehensive strategies that address multiple aspects of the malaria transmission cycle.

9.3.3 Community engagement and empowerment:

Engaging and empowering communities is crucial for sustainable malaria control. Successful interventions have shown that involving communities in decision-making, implementing interventions, and monitoring progress increases ownership and compliance. Future interventions should prioritize community engagement and empowerment, ensuring that communities are active participants in malaria control efforts.

9.3.4 Strong health systems:

Strong and resilient health systems are fundamental to effective malaria control. Success stories have highlighted the importance of strengthening health systems, including infrastructure, human resources, supply chains, and surveillance systems. Future interventions should prioritize health system strengthening to ensure sustainable and effective malaria control interventions.

9.3.5 Collaboration and partnerships:

Collaboration between governments, NGOs, the private sector, and international agencies is vital for successful malaria control. Success stories have demonstrated the power of partnerships in mobilizing resources, sharing expertise, and coordinating efforts. Future interventions should promote collaboration and partnerships at local, national, and international levels to leverage the strengths of different stakeholders.

9.3.6 Evidence-based decision-making:

Data-driven decision-making is critical for effective malaria control. Successful interventions have highlighted the importance of robust surveillance systems, accurate diagnostics, and monitoring and evaluation mechanisms. Future interventions should prioritize the collection and analysis of high-quality data to inform decision-making, monitor progress, and identify areas that require adjustments or targeted interventions.

9.3.7 Innovation and research:

Innovation plays a key role in malaria control. Successful interventions have embraced innovative approaches, technologies, and research to address challenges and improve outcomes. Future interventions should promote innovation, research, and development of new tools, strategies, and interventions to stay ahead of the evolving malaria landscape.

9.3.8 Regional collaboration and cross-border initiatives:

Malaria transmission does not respect borders, and regional collaboration is crucial. Success stories have emphasized the importance of regional collaboration and cross-border initiatives to address cross-border malaria transmission. Future interventions should promote collaboration between neighboring countries, harmonize strategies, and implement joint initiatives to effectively tackle malaria in border regions.

9.3.9 Sustainability and long-term commitment:

Malaria control is a long-term endeavor that requires sustained commitment. Success stories have highlighted the importance of sustained political commitment, predictable funding, and programmatic continuity. Future interventions should prioritize sustainability, secure long-term funding commitments, and ensure programmatic continuity to achieve and maintain malaria control and elimination goals.

By incorporating these lessons into future interventions, countries and regions can strengthen their malaria control efforts and move closer to achieving the goal of reducing the burden of malaria and ultimately eliminating the disease. Continuous learning, adaptation, and collaboration will be crucial to staying on track and addressing the evolving challenges in malaria control.

Chapter 10. Policy Implications and Recommendations

10.1 Discussion of policy implications based on the findings

The findings of the book on the impact of malaria on the socio-economic development of West Africa have several policy implications. These implications can guide policymakers in designing and implementing effective strategies to combat malaria and mitigate its negative consequences. The following are some key policy implications based on the findings:

10.1.1 Increased investment in malaria control:

The prevalence and burden of malaria in West Africa underscore the need for increased investment in malaria control efforts. Policymakers should prioritize allocating sufficient financial resources to malaria prevention, diagnosis, and treatment interventions. Adequate funding is necessary to ensure the availability and accessibility of essential tools and strategies, such as insecticide-treated bed nets, antimalarial drugs, and vector control measures.

10.1.2 Strengthened health systems:

Malaria control efforts can be enhanced by strengthening the health systems in West African countries. This includes improving infrastructure, increasing the number and training of healthcare workers, strengthening supply chains for essential medicines and diagnostics, and enhancing surveillance systems. A strong health system is vital for effective malaria control, as it ensures timely and accurate diagnosis, appropriate treatment, and efficient management of malaria cases.

10.1.3 Integrated approach to malaria control:

The book highlights the importance of a comprehensive and integrated approach to malaria control. Policymakers should prioritize the implementation of multi-faceted interventions that address different aspects of malaria transmission, such as vector control, case management, community engagement, and surveillance. Integrated approaches have been proven to be more effective in reducing malaria transmission and burden compared to single interventions alone.

10.1.4 Community engagement and empowerment:

Engaging and empowering communities is critical for the success of malaria control interventions. Policymakers should prioritize community involvement in decision-making, planning, and implementation of malaria control programs. This can be achieved through community education and awareness campaigns, mobilizing community resources, and promoting community-led initiatives. Empowered communities are more likely to adopt preventive measures, seek timely treatment, and actively participate in vector control activities.

Strengthened regional collaboration:

Malaria knows no boundaries, and regional collaboration is essential for effective control. Policymakers should promote collaboration between neighboring countries in West Africa to address cross-border malaria transmission. This can involve sharing information, harmonizing strategies, and implementing joint initiatives for surveillance, diagnosis, and treatment. Strengthened regional collaboration can help prevent the importation of malaria cases and ensure a coordinated response to the disease.

10.1.5 Continued research and innovation:

Policymakers should prioritize research and innovation in malaria control. This includes supporting research institutions and fostering partnerships between researchers, policymakers, and implementers. Investment in research can lead to the development of new tools, technologies, and strategies for malaria prevention, diagnosis, and treatment. Additionally, policymakers should encourage the adoption of innovative approaches, such as the use of new vector control methods and digital technologies for surveillance and monitoring.

10.1.6 Sustainable financing mechanisms:

Long-term sustainability of malaria control programs requires sustainable financing mechanisms. Policymakers should explore innovative financing mechanisms and ensure a predictable and adequate funding stream for malaria control activities. This can involve engaging with international donors, advocating for increased domestic funding, and exploring innovative financing mechanisms, such as social impact bonds or private sector partnerships.

10.1.7 Strengthened monitoring and evaluation systems:

Policymakers should prioritize the establishment and strengthening of robust monitoring and evaluation systems for malaria control programs. This includes regular data collection, analysis, and reporting to measure progress, identify gaps, and inform decision-making. Monitoring and evaluation systems are crucial for tracking the impact of interventions, identifying areas that require adjustment or scaling up, and ensuring accountability and transparency in malaria control efforts.

By considering these policy implications, policymakers can design and implement evidence-based strategies to combat malaria in West Africa. These strategies can contribute to reducing the prevalence and burden of malaria, mitigating its socio-economic impact

10.2 Recommendations for improving malaria control and prevention strategies in West Africa

Based on the findings of the book, the following recommendations are proposed to improve malaria control and prevention strategies in West Africa:

10.2.1 Strengthened surveillance and data systems:

Enhance the surveillance and data collection systems to improve the accuracy and timeliness of malaria information. This includes strengthening malaria case reporting, improving diagnostic capacity, and implementing real-time monitoring systems. Accurate and timely data are essential for targeted interventions, resource allocation, and monitoring progress.

10.2.2 Increased access to preventive measures:

Scale up the distribution and use of key preventive measures, such as insecticide-treated bed nets (ITNs) and indoor residual spraying (IRS). Ensure universal coverage of ITNs, particularly among vulnerable populations such as children and pregnant women. Intensify IRS campaigns in high-transmission areas to reduce mosquito populations and prevent malaria transmission.

10.2.3 Improved case management:

Enhance the quality and availability of diagnostic tools and antimalarial drugs to ensure accurate diagnosis and prompt treatment. Strengthen health worker capacity for early detection, diagnosis, and appropriate management of malaria cases. Implement quality assurance programs for diagnostic testing and treatment to improve the accuracy and effectiveness of case management.

10.2.4 Enhanced vector control strategies:

Explore and implement innovative vector control strategies to address insecticide resistance and improve control effectiveness. This may include the use of new insecticides, larval source management, biological control methods, and novel vector control technologies. Additionally, promote community participation in vector control efforts, such as environmental management and use of personal protective measures.

10.2.5 Community engagement and behavior change:

Empower communities through health education, community mobilization, and behavior change communication campaigns. Increase awareness about malaria prevention, early recognition of symptoms, and timely treatment-seeking behavior. Foster community ownership and participation in malaria control activities, including community-led surveillance, distribution of preventive measures, and environmental management.

10.2.6 Strengthened health systems:

Invest in strengthening health systems to ensure effective delivery of malaria control interventions. This includes improving infrastructure, increasing human resources, and strengthening supply chains for essential commodities. Enhance the capacity of healthcare workers through training programs on malaria diagnosis, treatment, and surveillance. Integrate malaria control efforts into existing primary healthcare systems to improve access and coverage.

10.2.7 Cross-sectoral collaboration:

Foster collaboration between the health sector and other relevant sectors, such as agriculture, education, and tourism. Integrate malaria control efforts with agricultural practices to minimize mosquito breeding sites. Promote malaria prevention and control education in schools and implement malaria control measures in tourist destinations. Collaboration across sectors can amplify the impact of malaria control efforts and contribute to sustainable development.

10.2.8 Research and innovation:

Prioritize research and innovation to develop new tools, technologies, and strategies for malaria control. Support research institutions and foster partnerships between researchers, policymakers, and implementers. Invest in operational research to evaluate the effectiveness of interventions, assess program impact, and identify best practices. Continuously monitor and adapt strategies based on emerging evidence and lessons learned.

10.2.9 Advocacy and resource mobilization:

Advocate for increased political commitment and resource mobilization for malaria control. Engage with policymakers, donors, and stakeholders to prioritize malaria on national and regional agendas. Strengthen partnerships with international donors, private sector organizations, and non-governmental organizations to secure sustained funding for malaria control programs.

10.2.10 Regional collaboration and knowledge sharing:

Facilitate regional collaboration and knowledge sharing among West African countries. Share experiences, lessons learned, and best practices to accelerate progress in malaria control. Collaborate on cross-border initiatives to address malaria transmission in border regions and minimize importation of cases.

By implementing these recommendations, West African countries can strengthen their malaria control and prevention strategies, reduce the burden of malaria, and contribute to improved socio-economic development in the region. Continuous monitoring, evaluation, and adaptation of strategies

10.3 Call for increased investment in research, healthcare infrastructure, and capacity building

To effectively combat malaria in West Africa and mitigate its impact on socio-economic development, there is a pressing need for increased investment in research, healthcare infrastructure, and capacity building. The following areas require specific attention:

10.3.1 Research:

Investment in malaria research is crucial for developing new tools, strategies, and interventions. There is a need to prioritize research on drug resistance, vector control, diagnostics, and vaccines. Funding research institutions, supporting collaborative research initiatives, and fostering partnerships between researchers, policymakers, and implementers will drive innovation and evidence-based decision-making.

10.3.2 Healthcare infrastructure:

Strengthening healthcare infrastructure is essential for the delivery of effective malaria control interventions. Investments should focus on improving healthcare facilities, expanding laboratory capacities, and enhancing the availability and accessibility of essential medicines, diagnostics, and equipment. Adequate infrastructure ensures timely diagnosis, appropriate treatment, and quality care for malaria patients.

10.3.3 Capacity building:

Building the capacity of healthcare workers, researchers, and public health professionals is vital for sustainable malaria control efforts. Investment should be directed towards training programs, workshops, and continuing education to enhance skills in malaria diagnosis, treatment, surveillance, and program management. Strengthening human resources in the health sector will contribute to the quality and effectiveness of malaria control interventions.

10.3.4 Surveillance systems:

Strengthening surveillance systems is crucial for monitoring the epidemiology and impact of malaria. Investments should be made to enhance data collection, analysis, and reporting, as well as the use of digital technologies for real-time monitoring. By improving surveillance systems, policymakers can make informed decisions, track progress, and identify areas that require targeted interventions.

10.3.5 Access to preventive measures and treatment:

Increased investment is needed to ensure universal access to preventive measures, such as insecticide-treated bed nets, and effective antimalarial drugs. This includes the procurement, distribution, and monitoring of the quality and effectiveness of these interventions. Adequate funding will help reduce financial barriers and ensure that vulnerable populations, such as children and pregnant women, have equitable access to preventive measures and treatment.

10.3.6 Health system strengthening:

Investment in health system strengthening is vital for effective malaria control. This includes improving infrastructure, supply chains, and laboratory capacities, as well as strengthening health workforce management and retention. A well-functioning health system ensures the delivery of integrated and quality healthcare services, contributing to better malaria control outcomes.

10.3.7 Collaborative partnerships:

Increased investment should be directed towards fostering collaborative partnerships between governments, NGOs, the private sector, and international agencies. Collaborative efforts can leverage expertise, resources, and innovative approaches for malaria control. Engaging stakeholders from multiple sectors will facilitate knowledge sharing, resource mobilization, and the implementation of comprehensive and coordinated interventions.

Investing in research, healthcare infrastructure, and capacity building will yield significant returns in the fight against malaria in West Africa. It will enable the development and implementation of evidence-based strategies, improve healthcare delivery, and ultimately reduce the burden of malaria on individuals, communities, and economies. Increased investment is not only a moral imperative but also an essential step towards achieving the goal of malaria elimination and sustainable development in the region.

Chapter 11. Conclusions

11.1 Summary of the main findings and key points discussed in the book

The book focused on the impact of malaria on the socio-economic development of West Africa. The main findings and key points discussed in the book are as follows:

Prevalence and burden of malaria: West Africa bears a significant burden of malaria, with high transmission rates and a large number of cases. The region accounts for a substantial proportion of global malaria cases and deaths, with children and pregnant women being particularly vulnerable.

Most affected countries and regions: Several countries in West Africa, such as Nigeria, Ghana, Burkina Faso, and Mali, experience a high prevalence of malaria. Certain regions within these countries, such as the Sahel region, face even higher transmission rates and increased malaria-related morbidity and mortality.

Factors contributing to high malaria transmission rates: West Africa's ecological and climatic conditions, including seasonal rainfall patterns and suitable breeding sites for mosquitoes, contribute to the high malaria transmission rates. Weak health systems, limited access to preventive measures and treatment, and socioeconomic factors further exacerbate the malaria burden.

Health consequences of malaria infection: Malaria infection leads to a range of health consequences, including fever, anemia, organ damage, and neurological complications. Severe malaria can result in hospitalization and death, particularly among children and pregnant women.

Impact on mortality rates: Malaria is a leading cause of mortality in West Africa, especially among children under five years old. Pregnant women are also at increased risk of severe complications and death due to malaria infection.

11.1.1 Long-term effects of repeated malaria infections:

Repeated malaria infections can have long-term effects on individuals' health and well-being. It can lead to chronic anemia, cognitive impairment, poor educational attainment, and reduced productivity in adulthood.

11.1.2 Productivity losses:

Malaria-related illnesses and deaths result in significant productivity losses in West Africa. The disease affects both individuals and the broader economy, leading to decreased agricultural productivity, absenteeism from work and school, and increased healthcare costs.

11.1.3 Impact on agriculture and food security:

Malaria has a detrimental impact on agriculture and food security in West Africa. It affects farming communities by reducing productivity, increasing labor absenteeism, and limiting access to nutritious food.

11.1.4 Healthcare costs and expenditures:

Malaria treatment and prevention impose a substantial financial burden on individuals, families, and healthcare systems. The costs include diagnostic tests, antimalarial drugs, hospitalization, and vector control measures.

11.1.5 Indirect costs:

Malaria has indirect costs that extend beyond the healthcare sector. It contributes to reduced educational attainment, as children miss school due to illness. Additionally, malaria can deter tourism, affecting the economies of countries reliant on tourism revenues.

Social consequences: Malaria can lead to stigma and discrimination against individuals and communities affected by the disease. The fear of transmission and misconceptions surrounding malaria can contribute to social exclusion and hinder community development.

Gender dimensions:

Malaria disproportionately affects women and girls in West Africa. Pregnant women are at higher risk of severe complications, and malaria can have adverse effects on maternal and child health outcomes. Gender disparities in access to healthcare and preventive measures further exacerbate the impact on women and girls.

11.1.6 Existing malaria control interventions:

West Africa has implemented various malaria control interventions, including vector control measures (such as bed nets and indoor spraying) and the use of antimalarial drugs. These interventions have shown effectiveness in reducing malaria transmission and improving health outcomes.

The book highlights challenges and limitations of current malaria control approaches, including insecticide resistance, limited access to healthcare services, inadequate funding, and weak health systems.

11.1.8 Innovative strategies:

The book discusses innovative strategies and technologies for malaria control, such as the use of new vector

11.2 Final remarks on the importance of addressing malaria as a critical factor in socio-economic development in West Africa

Addressing malaria in West Africa is of utmost importance for the region's socio-economic development. Malaria poses a significant burden on individuals, communities, and economies, hindering progress in various sectors. By prioritizing malaria control and prevention, West African countries can unlock substantial benefits and achieve sustainable development. The following points highlight the importance of addressing malaria as a critical factor in socio-economic development:

11.2.1 Health and well-being:

Malaria control is essential for improving the health and well-being of populations in West Africa. By reducing malaria-related morbidity and mortality, countries can enhance the overall health status of their citizens, leading to increased productivity and a better quality of life.

Malaria affects educational attainment, as children frequently miss school due to illness. By controlling malaria, countries can ensure that children have regular access to education, which is crucial for human capital development and long-term socio-economic growth.

11.2.3 Workforce productivity:

Malaria-related illnesses and deaths result in significant productivity losses in West Africa. By investing in malaria control, countries can reduce absenteeism, improve workforce productivity, and foster economic growth. A healthy workforce contributes to increased agricultural productivity, labor force participation, and overall economic development.

11.2.4 Poverty reduction:

Malaria perpetuates the cycle of poverty in West Africa. The disease primarily affects vulnerable populations and hampers their ability to escape poverty. By addressing malaria, countries can alleviate the economic burden on individuals and households, leading to poverty reduction and improved livelihoods.

11.2.5 Agriculture and food security:

Malaria impacts agricultural productivity and food security. By controlling malaria, countries can promote agricultural development, increase crop yields, and ensure food availability. This, in turn, enhances food security, reduces malnutrition, and supports economic resilience.

11.2.6 Tourism and economic diversification:

Malaria can deter tourism, an important source of revenue and employment in West Africa. By effectively controlling malaria, countries can attract more tourists, boost the tourism sector, and diversify their economies. A thriving tourism industry contributes to job creation, foreign exchange earnings, and local economic development.

11.2.7 Regional cooperation and integration:

Addressing malaria requires regional cooperation and integration efforts. West African countries share common challenges and can benefit from joint initiatives, knowledge sharing, and resource pooling. Collaborative approaches foster regional stability, strengthen health systems, and promote sustainable development across borders.

11.2.8 Sustainable development goals:

Tackling malaria aligns with the United Nations' Sustainable Development Goals (SDGs). Malaria control contributes to achieving SDG 3 (Good Health and Well-being) by reducing malaria-related morbidity and mortality. It also supports SDG 1 (No Poverty), SDG 2 (Zero Hunger), and SDG 4 (Quality Education) by improving socio-economic conditions and fostering human development.

In conclusion, addressing malaria as a critical factor in socio-economic development is paramount for West Africa. By prioritizing and investing in malaria control and prevention, countries can improve health outcomes, enhance educational opportunities, increase workforce productivity, reduce poverty, ensure food security, stimulate economic growth, and advance progress towards sustainable development goals. A comprehensive and multi-sectoral approach is needed, involving collaboration between governments, NGOs, the private sector, and international agencies. The successful control of malaria will contribute to a healthier, more prosperous, and resilient West Africa.

11.3 Appendices

252

11.3.1 Keywords:

Absenteeism: The act of being absent from work, school, or other responsibilities.

Acute Respiratory Distress Syndrome (ARDS): A severe lung condition that leads to rapid onset respiratory failure.

Anemia: A condition characterized by a decrease in the number of red blood cells or a lower than normal level of hemoglobin in the blood.

Antimalarial Treatments: Medications used to treat malaria infections and alleviate its symptoms.

Cerebral Malaria: A severe complication of malaria characterized by the infection of the brain by malaria parasites.

Cognitive Development: The process of acquiring knowledge, understanding, and problem-solving abilities as individuals grow and mature.

Cognitive Impairments: Difficulties and deficits in cognitive functions, such as memory, attention, and learning, resulting from malaria infections.

Community Development: Efforts to improve the well-being and living conditions of a community through various initiatives and projects.

Community Empowerment: Efforts to enhance the capacity of individuals and communities to participate in decision-making and improve their well-being.

Community Engagement: Involving community members in activities, decisions, and initiatives that affect their well-being and development.

Community Participation: The involvement of community members in decision-making processes and activities that affect their well-being and development.

Diagnostic Tools: Medical equipment or tests used to detect and diagnose malaria infections.

Economic Burden: The financial costs and losses associated with malaria infections, including healthcare expenses and reduced productivity.

Endemic Regions: Geographic areas where malaria is regularly and consistently present and transmitted.

Equitable Access: Ensuring fair and equal access to resources and opportunities for all individuals and communities.

Healthcare Expenditures: The costs associated with healthcare services, treatments, and medications.

Hemoglobin: The protein in red blood cells that carries oxygen from the lungs to the body's tissues.

Indoor Residual Spraying (IRS): A vector control strategy that involves applying insecticides to the interior walls of houses to kill mosquitoes that rest on these surfaces.

Insecticide-Treated Bed Nets (ITNs): Bed nets that are treated with insecticides to repel or kill mosquitoes that come into contact with them, providing protection against malaria transmission during sleep.

Local Governance: The administration and decision-making processes at the local community or government level.

Malaria: A mosquito-borne infectious disease caused by Plasmodium parasites, transmitted to humans through the bites of infected female Anopheles mosquitoes.

Multi-organ Failure: The failure of multiple organ systems in the body.

Multi-Organizational Collaboration: Collaboration between multiple organizations and entities to address malaria control and related challenges.

Multi-sectoral Approach: An approach that involves collaboration and coordination between multiple sectors or disciplines to address complex issues like malaria control.

Participatory Decision-Making: Involving all relevant stakeholders in the decision-making process to ensure diverse perspectives are considered.

Productivity Losses: The reduction in work capacity and output due to malaria-related illnesses, leading to decreased economic productivity.

Prompt Diagnosis: The timely identification of malaria cases to initiate appropriate treatment promptly.

Research and Development: Efforts to explore new interventions, technologies, and strategies for addressing malaria and related challenges.

Severe Malaria: A severe and life-threatening form of malaria that can lead to organ failure and other complications.

Social Cohesion: The degree to which individuals in a community or society work together and form strong social bonds.

Social Inequalities: Disparities and differences in social and economic status among individuals and communities.

Socio-economic Development: The improvement of social and economic conditions in a community or society.

Stigma: Negative perceptions or attitudes towards individuals or groups due to certain characteristics or conditions, such as having malaria.

Sustainable Development: Development that meets the needs of the present without compromising the ability of future generations to meet their needs.

Vector Control: Strategies aimed at controlling the population and transmission of disease-carrying vectors, such as mosquitoes.

Ahorlu, C. K., et al. (2019). Community factors influencing uptake of intermittent preventive treatment for malaria in pregnancy in the context of a clustered randomized trial in Ghana. Malaria Journal, 18(1).

Alout, H., et al. (2014). Impact of insecticide resistance alleles on susceptibility to the synergistic effects of pyrethroid-organophosphate mixtures in the malaria vector Anopheles gambiae. PLoS One, 9(4), e96250.

Bogoch, I. I., Utzinger, J., Lo, N. C., Andrews, J. R., & Qi, J. (2020). Malaria hotspot areas in a highland Kenya site are consistent spatially and temporally.

Brooker, S., et al. (2000). Epidemiology of Plasmodium-helminth co-infection in Africa: populations at risk, potential impact on anemia, and prospects for combining control. The American Journal of Tropical Medicine and Hygiene, 77(6_Suppl), 88-98.

Chima, R. I., Goodman, C. A., Mills, A. (2010). The economic impact of malaria in Africa: a critical review of the evidence. Health Policy, 63(1), 17-36.

Chuma, J., Gilson, L., Molyneux, C. (2006). Treatment-seeking behaviour, cost burdens and coping strategies among rural and urban households in Coastal Kenya: an equity analysis. Tropical Medicine & International Health, 11(5), 673-686.

Deressa, W., et al. (2017). Community participation and involvement in malaria control: an evidence-based review. Malaria Journal, 16(1), 1-11.

Desai, M., ter Kuile, F. O., Nosten, F., McGready, R., Asamoa, K., Brabin, B., ... & Newman, R. D. (2018). Epidemiology and burden of malaria in pregnancy. The Lancet Infectious Diseases, 7(2), 93-104.

Ettling, M. B., et al. (1992). The economic impact of malaria in Africa: a critical review of the evidence.

Fernando, S. D., Rodrigo, C., Rajapakse, S. (2016). The 'hidden' burden of malaria: cognitive impairment following infection. Malaria Journal, 15(1), 285.

Fillinger, U., et al. (2009). The practical importance of permanent and semipermanent habitats for controlling aquatic stages of Anopheles gambiae sensu lato mosquitoes: operational observations from a rural town in western Kenya. Tropical Medicine & International Health, 14(5), 506-515.

Gallup, J. L., & Sachs, J. D. (2001). The economic burden of malaria. American Journal of Tropical Medicine and Hygiene, 64(1_suppl), 85-96.

Gething, P. W., Casey, D. C., Weiss, D. J., Bisanzio, D., Bhatt, S., Cameron, E., ... & Moyes, C. L. (2016). Mapping Plasmodium falciparum mortality in Africa between 1990 and 2015. New England Journal of Medicine, 375(25), 2435-2445.

Global Fund. (n.d.). Malaria. Retrieved from https://www.theglobalfund.org/en/malaria/

Koenker, H., et al. (2016). Assessing whether malaria control interventions have a net impact on entomological indices in an area of intense transmission: a pilot evaluation in southwestern Uganda. Malaria Journal, 15(1), 420.

Lengeler, C. (2004). Insecticide-treated bed nets and curtains for preventing malaria. Cochrane Database of Systematic Reviews, (2), CD000363.

Littrell, M., S. et al. (2013). Impact of a malaria control program on household expenditures: a case study from rural Zambia. Malaria Journal, 12(1), 46.

Noland, G. S., Graves, P. M., Sallau, A., Eigege, A., Emukah, E., Patterson, A. E., ... & Obiezu, J. (2020). Malaria prevalence, anemia and baseline intervention coverage prior to mass net distributions in Abia and Plateau States, Nigeria. BMC Infectious Diseases, 20(1), 1-14.

Okumu, F. O., et al. (2010). Indoor residual spraying with alphacypermethrin controls malaria in a holoendemic region of Tanzania where bed nets alone had a modest impact on transmission. Malaria Journal, 9(1), 1-14.

O'Meara, W. P., Mangeni, J. N., Steketee, R., & Greenwood, B. (2010). Changes in the burden of malaria in sub-Saharan Africa. The Lancet Infectious Diseases, 10(8), 545-555.

Pennetier, C., et al. (2013). Synergy between repellents and organophosphates on bed nets: efficacy and behavioural response of natural free-flying An. gambiae mosquitoes. PLoS One, 8(12), e80694.

Ranson, H., et al. (2011). Pyrethroid resistance in African anopheline mosquitoes: what are the implications for malaria control? Trends in Parasitology, 27(2), 91-98.

RBM Partnership. (n.d.). West Africa. Retrieved from https://endmalaria.org/region/west-africa

Rénia, L., Howland, S. W., & Claser, C. (2018). Cerebral malaria: mysteries at the blood–brain barrier. Virulence, 9(1), 1668-1690.

Sachs, J., & Malaney, P. (2002). The economic and social burden of malaria. Nature, 415(6872), 680-685.

Strode, C., et al. (2014). Contemporary insecticide resistance: Leaps and bounds to overcome. Trends in Parasitology, 30(6), 271-280.

Tusting, L. S., Bisanzio, D., Alabaster, G., Cameron, E., Cibulskis, R., Davies, M., ... & Gething, P. W. (2020). Mapping changes in housing in sub-Saharan Africa from 2000 to 2015. Nature, 585(7823), 398-402.

West Africa. Retrieved from https://www.pmi.gov/where-we-work/west-africa

World Health Organization (WHO). (2019). World malaria report 2019. Retrieved from https://www.who.int/publications/i/item/world-malaria-report-2019

World Health Organization. (2020). World Malaria Report 2020. Retrieved from https://www.who.int/publications/i/item/9789240015791

Don't miss out!

Visit the website below and you can sign up to receive emails whenever Mogana S. Flomo, Jr. publishes a new book. There's no charge and no obligation.

https://books2read.com/r/B-A-JCHY-BYVLC

BOOKS2READ

Connecting independent readers to independent writers.

About the Author

Dr. Mogana S. Flomo, Jr. is a highly accomplished and versatile individual, with expertise in several fields including education, agriculture, public health, and social sector leadership. He was born on February 13, 1976, in Jorwah, Panta District, Bong County, Republic of Liberia, to Prof. and Mrs. Mogana S. Flomo, Sr.

Dr. Flomo is the Founder of the Center for Environmental and Public Health Research (CEPRES) Inc. and CEPRES International University in Liberia. He has over 25 years of experience in teaching at various universities in Liberia, including Cuttington University, Bong County Technical College, and CEPRES International University. Dr. Flomo currently serves as a Special Technical Consultant to the National Commission on Higher Education and is the immediate Former Minister of Agriculture of the Republic of Liberia.

Apart from his roles in education and agriculture, Dr. Flomo is also involved in politics and public service. He has served as Board Chairman and member of many organizations, institutions, and agencies of government, including Youth for Positive Transformation Initiative (YOPTI), Liberia Initiative for Developmental Services (LIDS), National Public Health Institute of Liberia (NPHIL), National Fisheries and Aquaculture Authority (NaFAA), Central Agriculture Research Institute (CARI), Forestry Development Authority (FDA) of Liberia, Booker Washington Institute, Liberia Bank for Development and Investment (LBDI), and several others.

Dr. Flomo is an accomplished author with several publications in health, education, and agriculture, as well as a book on Decision Making. He is the Head of the Africa Mission of the International Academic and Management Association (IAMA), headquartered in Delhi, India.

Dr. Flomo's passion for human development is evident in his work and involvement in youth-focused initiatives. He has worked extensively with communities, including farming groups in rural

Liberia, for more than ten years. Dr. Flomo is also an environmentalist and a public health professional with a keen interest in improving Liberia's food security and education system.

Dr. Flomo is an expert in several software programs, including Statistics Software (STATA, Python, and R), Music Software (Cakewalk Pro-audio, Cakewalk Sonar Producer Edition, and more), and has excellent skills in setting up and managing several Distance Education Platforms.

www.ingramcontent.com/pod-product-compliance
Lightning Source LLC
Chambersburg PA
CBHW021147160726
47994CB00001B/115